# ✚ EMERGENCIES ONLY

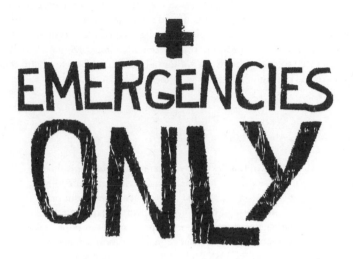

# EMERGENCIES ONLY

AN AUSTRALIAN NURSE'S JOURNEY THROUGH
NATURAL DISASTERS, EXTREME POVERTY,
CIVIL WARS AND GENERAL CHAOS

## AMANDA McCLELLAND
WITH SIMONE UBALDI

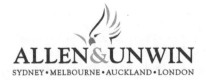

ALLEN&UNWIN
SYDNEY·MELBOURNE·AUCKLAND·LONDON

Certain names and details have been changed to protect the innocent and guilty alike.

The author confirms that the views and opinions expressed in this publication are entirely her own and do not in any way constitute the official view or position of the International Federation of the Red Cross & Red Crescent, the International Committee of the Red Cross, Concern Worldwide, or any other organisation mentioned within this book. Every effort has been made to comply with the author's obligation of discretion with regard to activities undertaken during her missions with these organisations.

First published in 2017

Allen & Unwin
83 Alexander Street
Crows Nest NSW 2065
Australia
Phone:    (61 2) 8425 0100
Email:    info@allenandunwin.com
Web:      www.allenandunwin.com

Cataloguing-in-Publication details are available
from the National Library of Australia
www.trove.nla.gov.au

ISBN 978 1 76029 421 2

Map by Romina Panetta
Set in 13/17 pt Bembo by Midland Typesetters, Australia
Printed and bound in Australia by Griffin Press

10 9 8 7 6 5 4 3 2

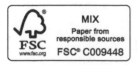

# Contents

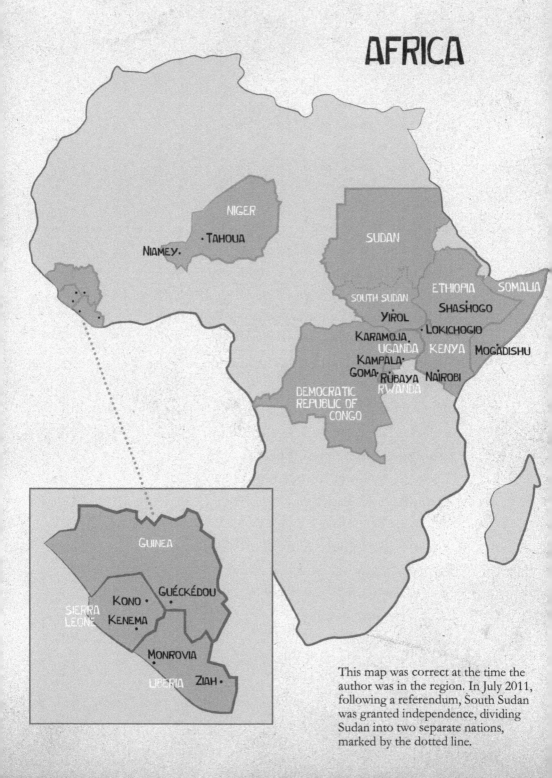

GENEVA, SWITZERLAND

# AFRICA

NIGER

• TAHOUA

NIAMEY •

SUDAN

ETHIOPIA

SOMALIA

SOUTH SUDAN

SHASHOGO

YIROL •

• LOKICHOGIO

KARAMOJA •

KENYA

UGANDA

MOGADISHU

KAMPALA •

GOMA • RUBAYA • NAIROBI

RWANDA

DEMOCRATIC
REPUBLIC OF
CONGO

GUINEA

GUÉCKÉDOU

KONO •

SIERRA
LEONE

KENEMA

MONROVIA •

ZIAH •

LIBERIA

This map was correct at the time the
author was in the region. In July 2011,
following a referendum, South Sudan
was granted independence, dividing
Sudan into two separate nations,
marked by the dotted line.

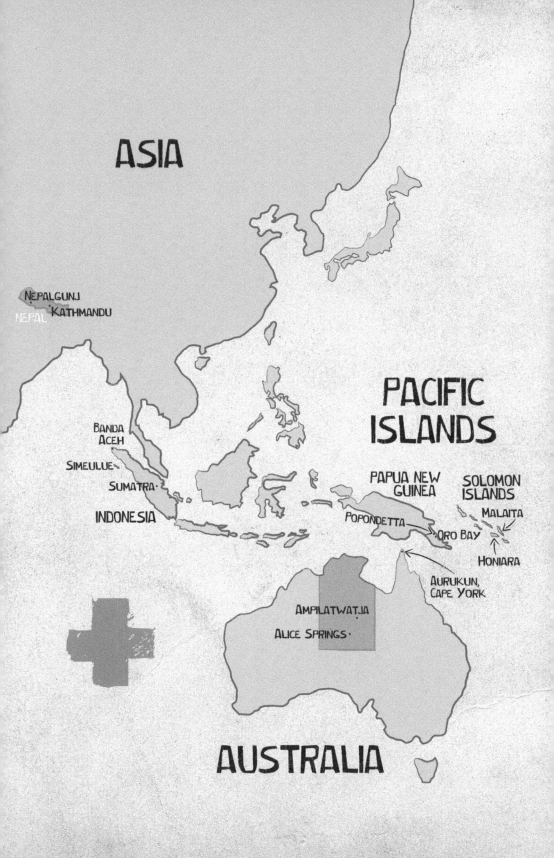

ASIA

NEPALGUNJ
NEPAL · KATHMANDU

PACIFIC
ISLANDS

BANDA
ACEH

SIMEULUE

SUMATRA ·

INDONESIA

PAPUA NEW
GUINEA

POPONDETTA

ORO BAY

SOLOMON
ISLANDS

MALAITA

HONIARA

AURUKUN,
CAPE YORK

AMPILATWATJA

ALICE SPRINGS ·

AUSTRALIA

'When are you going to get a real life?'

My sister gestured broadly at the 'real life' around her. We were sitting in the lounge room of her beautiful Queenslander home, which has an actual picket fence out the front and a kidney-shaped pool in the backyard. There was a 50-centimetre television right behind my sister, her SUV was parked in the driveway, and in one of the many bedrooms, her child was having a nap.

I don't have any of these things—no big house in suburbia, no big car, no swimming pool and no kids—but there's a very good reason for that. I've spent the better part of twenty years in the field, doing humanitarian aid work. I've worked in civil war, famine, tsunami and disease epidemics, and I've had quite a good time doing it. My job *is* real life, as far as I'm concerned. It's just a little different from hers.

# 1

# A TOWN LIKE ALICE

There is one road in and out of Alice Springs and it runs 1500 kilometres in either direction. Smack bang in the middle of the Stuart Highway, surrounded by red desert, Alice is a squat and dusty little town. It has palm trees, scrub and bone-dry streets, a few pubs and a parched football ground. At four storeys, the Alice Springs Hospital is the tallest building in town—at least it was when I arrived. I was twenty-one years old, a newly qualified nurse. Alice was the beginning.

I hadn't dreamed of becoming a nurse. I hadn't pictured myself dressing wounds and changing bedpans by lamplight, with a little red cross embroidered over my heart. I thought I might be a cartoonist, or maybe a teacher. I had seriously considered joining the police force, but my mother talked me out of it. She was convinced I wouldn't get to have a family if I signed up—I think she assumed that all female police officers had to take a vow of celibacy. If I was a nurse I could have kids, my mother reasoned. I was going to disappoint her there.

Mum was a nurse's aide, and later a phlebotomist. She always thought I would do something to help people because I was very community-minded, but I took to nursing because it was interesting, not because I was on some mission to make the world a better place. I started the degree initially because I didn't get the points for physiotherapy, figuring I would transfer across later in the program. But nursing turned out to be so diverse and interesting, I didn't want to leave.

During the three-year course, we did a number of different work placements so that we could learn the vital practical aspects of the job and get a feel for the different areas of healthcare. I spent some time in a family planning clinic in the red-light district of Brisbane, listening to qualified nurses counsel pregnant teenagers and treat sexual health problems. It taught me a lot about the importance of communication (and gave me a paralysing fear of STDs). My next placement was in a psychiatric care facility, where a very pleasant man, wearing nothing but a nappy, chatted to me about the joys of drinking coffee from a baby's bottle. Later I spent some time in a nursing home where, at the age of eighteen, I gave my first sponge bath to an elderly gentleman. I giggled uncontrollably at the time but those awkward physical encounters were soon just another part of the job.

My final work placement was at the Royal Children's Hospital in Brisbane, a bright building with cartoon characters painted on the walls. I knew almost as soon as I started that I wanted to be a paediatric nurse. Kids made for interesting patients. Adults are fairly robust; they're better able to cope if you make a mistake with medication or observations, and they can tell you if they don't feel right. Children are less likely to communicate that something's going wrong, and when they crash, they crash fast. The margin of error with children is really small, and for me that represented a real challenge. There was a lot of joy in it, too. I studied hard, but I also spent a lot of time making balloon animals from rubber gloves and playing PlayStation with my patients. I thought paediatric nursing was cool.

Early in my placement, I was assigned to an orthopaedic ward where a toddler had had a full hindquarter amputation: he'd lost one of his legs from the hip. He had just come out of the operating theatre, so the mood in the ward was very serious, and the clinical nurse asked me to continue his post-operative observations while the team met with the parents to discuss the rehabilitation strategy. The kid would have to relearn how to roll over, sit up and, eventually, how to walk. There was a long, difficult road ahead.

The thing is, when I got to his ward, the little boy was already on his feet (or foot, as it were). He was standing up, peering out between the bars of his cot, wondering where everyone had gone. He sat down with a bump when I walked in, happy as anything. *Good job, kid*, I smiled. The room next door was full of specialists worrying about how they were going to realign his balance and get him mobile again, but the little boy had figured it out for himself in about five minutes. The biggest problem we had all day was trying to keep a nappy on a one-legged toddler without having to use gaffer tape.

I had an epiphany. I realised I liked working with kids because they're so resilient; they bounce back quickly. And because we saw such great results, the work was really satisfying. I became quite addicted to that feeling during my career. Some people work their whole lives to achieve small, incremental changes, but that isn't my style. When it comes to making an impact, I prefer things fast and dramatic.

When I finished my degree, I was offered a graduate position at the Royal Children's and continued working there for the next eighteen months. I was lucky to be offered the position and I loved the job, but I knew I didn't want to spend my entire career working at the same hospital. It bothered me that many of the senior nurses there had never worked anywhere else.

Some of the younger nurses were talking about moving to London for a year—there was virtually an exchange program between the Royal Children's Hospital in Brisbane and Great Ormond Street Hospital in London—but I knew that wasn't for me. I didn't want to live in a congested European city, drinking and partying every weekend. I wanted to see more of Australia before I went overseas.

One day, a little Aboriginal girl from the south of Queensland was brought into the hospital with severe burns to her groin and bottom. She had pulled a pot of boiling water off the stove, spilling it all over her little body, and while the family had taken her straight to the bathroom to run her under cold water, they hadn't thought to take off her nappy. The water had pooled under the plastic sheath and burned her severely, leaving livid pink wounds on her.

The paediatric burns unit at the Royal Children's relied heavily on the parents' support when they treated babies. When a child had severe burns, the nurses would bathe it and use the water to slough off the dead epidermis. The child was sedated, of course, but it was still incredibly painful, and the parents were expected to be there to help the kid get through it. The mother of this little girl hadn't been there for the bath, for some reason. I heard the other nurses muttering about it; they were dumbfounded. The mother hadn't been there much at all since the child was admitted.

When the mum did come in, she looked frightened and lost. There was an Aboriginal liaison officer on the ward, but she didn't seem to understand any better than the nursing staff what had gone wrong, or where the woman had been. The liaison officer asked her why she hadn't used the taxi voucher she'd been given, but the mother had had no idea how to call a taxi. They'd given her an ATM card, but she had never used one before. The woman hadn't eaten, because she didn't know where to get food. She was too afraid to go into the supermarket. In ways we couldn't begin to understand, she was completely overwhelmed by the city. I didn't quite know what to make of it, but it didn't seem right.

A week or so after I'd had this encounter, I came across a job advertisement for the hospital in Alice Springs. It was a paediatric nursing role working in Aboriginal health, in the dead centre of the country, servicing a small community in the desert, roughly three thousand kilometres from Brisbane along vast stretches of sunburnt roads. I thought of that little Aboriginal girl and her mother, wondering if there was something I could learn that would have improved their experience. I liked the idea of working in the outback. The timing was great—I had just bought a four-wheel drive.

Getting to Alice Springs was an adventure, the first of many. After two days of solid driving, the car broke down just outside of Julia Creek. I had to wait a whole weekend for the spare part to come in, eating sausage rolls from the one petrol station in town and fending off the advances of Julia Creek's drunk ringers. I hadn't planned on the delay and didn't want to be late for my first day of work, so when I hit the road again, I took a short cut to try to make up the lost time. I ended up on a very, very long stretch of groomed dirt road between Julia Creek and nowhere. Not long after sunrise, I got sideswiped by a seven-foot kangaroo. The roo gave me a dirty look but hopped away unscathed, leaving a massive dent in my rear wheel guard. I sliced my hand open trying to fix it, then got bogged in a torrential rainstorm and was stuck on that lonely highway until two grey nomads came to the rescue. Anyway, long story short, I *was* late for my first day of work. I turned up at the Alice Springs Hospital covered head to toe in mud and blood, a large bandage around my hand, my car caked in red desert dust. Alice was a rogue town, though. No one batted an eyelid.

I was assigned to Ward 4 of the Alice Springs Hospital, the infectious paediatric unit. The ward looked much the same as the infectious paediatric unit in Brisbane, if a little less high-tech. We dealt with a fair amount of meningitis in the unit, but the biggest paediatric health issue in Alice Springs was diarrhoea. Working in Aboriginal paediatric health meant being up to my elbows in poo.

Most of the kids who came in from remote communities around Alice were under two years old. We grouped them together based on different strains of bacterial, parasitic or viral infection—shigella, giardia, campylobacter. We had to keep the giardia kids separate from the shigella kids because they'd infect each other and end up with two different bugs, and two different types of diarrhoea. I learned pretty quickly to distinguish different bacterial infections based on the colour, texture and the smell of a kid's poo—frothy, green or sickly sweet—because each strain of diarrhoea had its own unique character. Once I'd been in Alice for a while, I was able to triage the kids just by changing their nappies.

It turned out that nappy changing was a big part of the job. In fact, the greatest challenge I faced in the first few weeks was learning how to put on a cloth nappy so that liquid stool wouldn't leak out, though my technique was never foolproof. The whole team wore surgical scrubs because they were easy to replace when they got splattered with shit. The ward smelled kind of funky, but I got used to it.

The Aboriginal kids were gorgeous. They were used to being cared for by a whole community of people, so they were very easygoing. They didn't fuss when you picked them up or when their mums weren't around, and they didn't need your undivided attention, but caring for them was a much bigger part of the job than it had been in Brisbane. The cultural environment was very different, which meant the kids were left with us for significant chunks of time, and we were responsible for their general care as well as technical nursing. I spent a lot of time with a child on each hip and another one trailing at my feet—a six-foot-two Mary Poppins in Blundstone boots and scrubs.

The carers came in and out of the ward during the day in between other business. They lived in communities well outside of town and some of them had never been to Alice Springs before. In between hospital visits, they would spend time with family, or head to the local Kmart to buy their kid new clothes, so the kids were often better dressed when they left than when they came in. Some of the mothers would go down to the dry riverbed that runs through Alice to hang out with the local mob and drink, but they would all find their way back to the hospital eventually.

At night, we'd lay mattresses on the floor and take the babies out of their cots so that they could sleep next to their mothers the way that they did at home. The mothers would sleep with their hospital gowns unbuttoned to the waist, their breasts exposed so that their babies could latch on in the night whenever they needed to feed. The whole set-up was a little unorthodox, but it made sense for the families in our care. We worked around the obstacles. I still had to do observation checks every two hours regardless of where the kids were sleeping, so I spent quite a few nights scuttling between mattresses on my knees, looking for little patients in the dark.

They say that if you see the river run through Alice three times, you'll never leave town. The permanent staff at the hospital were stuck that way. They just loved the desert. They kept themselves slightly apart from the temporary staff; they weren't unfriendly, but used to seeing people come and go. The rest of us were clumped together in communal housing, sleeping and eating beside each other, looking for novel ways to kill time between shifts. There wasn't much in the way of entertainment in Alice except for the pub and the pool in the nurses' quarters. There was no internet, except at the local library, where it ran at some prehistoric dial-up speed. There may have been a ping pong table in the common room.

It was my first experience living and working with people who were far from home. It was a diverse group, but we all had one thing in common: we were searching for something we couldn't find in the suburbs. The money was good in Alice, but it was more than that. We all wanted to lead unusual lives. At least I think that's what was going on—it was for me. Why else would you move to a scratched-out town in the middle of nowhere?

The bush lifestyle suited me, especially the camping. We'd often jump in the car at the end of a shift, drive out into the scrub and sleep out overnight, then head back in the morning in time for work, getting lost temporarily in the landscape. Uluru was on our doorstep and it was magical—a hulking bit of grandeur in the desert.

We went four-wheel driving and mountain biking, exploring the different corners of the bush, and we drank a lot of beer, as you do. I've always been the outdoor type, and I'm quite partial to beer. Getting drunk under the Milky Way was not a bad way to spend an evening.

As the weeks rolled into months in Alice Springs, I started seeing the same faces coming through the ward again and again, a cohort of ten or fifteen kids who were almost constantly sick. Along with the gastro, they had scabies and ear infections. They were severely dehydrated and some of them had potassium levels that were barely life-sustaining, which blew my mind. A white kid in Brisbane with similar bloodwork would be in intensive care, but the Aboriginal children were able to survive with very low haemoglobin and potassium levels because the reduction had been gradual over time and consistent. Their bodies had adapted to being continually sick. They seemed to have a higher tolerance for pain, like their parents. They could endure the desert heat without problems, and their bodies had found a way to function despite being chronically under threat. Having to endure poor health conditions for such a long time had made them really robust, in a weird way, but by normal Western measures they were in serious trouble.

The kids were underweight, smaller than they should have been, and a lot of their developmental milestones were delayed. Later in my career, I would have recognised it as malnutrition, but we didn't call it that in Alice. We called it 'failure to thrive', which was an interesting diagnosis: it completely sidestepped the issue. It pointed out the effects of the problem, without looking for the source.

Seeing the same kids over and over again bothered me. I asked a lot of questions, especially early on, but I didn't really have a clear picture of what was happening from a public health perspective.

I was a clinical nurse at the beginning of my career and I had little awareness about public health. I had an intuition that there was some kind of systemic problem in the community, but my job was to treat kids when they got to hospital. I wasn't trained to think about the problem any other way.

I learned later that children in the Aboriginal communities around Alice usually ate when the rest of the family ate, though preschool kids need food or snacks four or five times a day. In some of the more remote areas it was hard to find clean water, let alone nutritious food like fruits and vegetables, which compounded the problem. Many of the kids had diarrhoea so often that their bowels were damaged and they couldn't absorb nutrients properly. Their guts took a while to heal and by then they usually had another bout of gastro, which weakened them even further. On top of everything else, being malnourished made them constantly susceptible to other kinds of infection, like meningitis and pneumonia, and over-crowding in the Aboriginal communities meant that infections spread quickly. The whole thing was a vicious cycle, happening largely out of view.

I didn't know back then how much a lack of basic hygiene played a role in their poor health. Not once did I speak to one of their mothers about regular handwashing, for example, or how to ensure their child had adequate nutrition. I was a nurse and this was the community I was supposed to care for, but it just wasn't part of the program. It was extraordinary to realise later that the major health crises we were battling in the developing world were going untreated in our own backyard.

We had a baby come into the ward one day who was in a serious condition, but we had no idea what was wrong with him. He would stop breathing for no reason and turn cyanotic blue—the colour of his skin was just incredible. We couldn't keep the apnoea monitors on him when he was awake because he was so small, so the nurses took turns carrying him around the ward, rubbing his chest whenever his colour turned and trying to stimulate his breathing. I carried that kid around through three different shifts, hoping he wouldn't die in my arms.

While all of this was going on, the baby's mother left the hospital. We had no idea if she was scared or angry, we just knew she was gone. The Aboriginal health worker on the ward didn't seem fussed, but then she rarely seemed fussed about anything. She was a solid old lady with tiny legs and a tiny bum but a massive round belly, relaxed and unflappable—our link to the community. Technically, she was supposed to help us care for the kids, but good luck getting her to change a nappy. She was invaluable when it came to managing the young mums, though; we wouldn't have had a clue otherwise. The old health worker told us the mother would be back, though she didn't know or couldn't tell us when.

When the mother returned, she brought a Ngangkari with her—a traditional healer from her tribe. They had been out to their tribal lands to dig up the woman's placenta and had come back to the hospital with a piece of the baby's umbilical cord wrapped in a cloth. The Ngangkari pinned the umbilical cord to the little white singlet the baby was wearing and the Aboriginal health worker told us he would be fine. Seemed unlikely to me, but by then I'd seen a few things at the hospital that I couldn't explain. We convinced the baby's mother to stick around for a few more days, just in case, but whatever had been wrong was right all of a sudden and our doctors didn't know why. I carried the baby around for another two or three shifts, but he didn't turn blue again.

The Aboriginal healthcare workers at Alice Springs Hospital kept a store of pituri in the adult ward, a bush chewing tobacco with nicotine-like properties, for patients who were at risk of going into withdrawal. When the hospital supply of pituri ran out, the old health worker on my ward offered to take me out to show me where they find it. She knew I was curious about her culture because I asked a lot of questions, and I jumped at the chance. I even convinced my friend Anthea to come along.

The health worker lived in a besser-block house in a community half an hour outside Alice. Anthea and I packed a picnic lunch and set off early to pick her up, knowing the heat would skyrocket as the summer day went on. When we arrived, the old health worker came out with two young nieces in tow, all three of them piling in beside us in my two-door Feroza, five bodies squeezed onto one long seat, with the sun climbing overhead.

The drive was a bit longer than expected. We were on one of those dead straight highways where the horizon is so wide you can see the curve of the earth. Then suddenly, out of nowhere, a goanna shot out in front of the car. I swerved to avoid it, but the old health worker shrieked and pounded on the back of my head, motioning for me to stop, so I slammed on the brakes. She was scrambling over me to get out of the door before the car had stopped moving, off like a shot into the bush, chasing after the goanna. The woman moved like a snail at the hospital, so I was pretty impressed. Unfortunately, she wasn't fast enough to catch her prey. She wandered barefoot and empty-handed out of the scrub, cursing my name. 'Next time, you run over it!' she told me. 'And when you run over it, run over the head. The tail is the bit that tastes good.'

An hour further along the road, the health worker gestured for us to stop and we all got out to hunt for the pituri plant. The old woman was very smart; she took the shady side of the road and sent Anthea and me to search on the sunny side. When we came back with nothing, after a good hour of searching, she told us the plant doesn't really like to grow in the sun, but it was good to check anyway.

While we had been away, the old lady and her nieces had eaten all the food we'd brought for lunch and polished off most of the water. It was past midday and the mercury was soaring, getting close to 45 degrees Celsius. 'At least we've got the pituri,' I comforted Anthea. 'We can head back.'

'Not yet,' our guide told us. 'We need the tree.'

Pituri is made by mixing the plant with wood ash from the bark of a particular bush tree. We still had to find the tree, or no pituri. *Ah for fuck's sake*, I thought. I was sweating bullets, but I remained committed to the operation.

For the next hour or so, we drove through the bush pointing at trees while the old woman shook her head, *no*. When we finally found the tree she wanted, she made me climb it to get the bark. I was dank and dehydrated, and halfway up the trunk it occurred to me to wonder why I'd been sent up there instead of one of the nieces. Just as I looked down to ask them, the two girls and their auntie disappeared. They had shot off into the bush again and were calling for me and Anthea to follow. One of them had spotted an echidna burrow and they were all very excited about the prospect of eating echidna for dinner. For the next forty-five minutes, the old health worker sat by as we dug into the hole trying to catch her meal, but the spiky little thing was too fast for us and it managed to get away. We did find a nest of honey ants nearby, so we took those home instead.

By the time we got back to the health worker's house, Anthea and I were dying of the heat. The old lady invited us in for a cup of tea and we said yes, though we were filthy and exhausted, and dying to join our mates back at the nurses' quarters for a swim. There was no polite way to say no, but in the end I was glad we stayed. The old woman squeezed the honey ants into the tea and it tasted lovely.

Later, our work colleagues told us that the pituri hunt was a bit of a hospital tradition. The old health worker had led a few people into the bush on a wild goose chase, eating the picnic lunch, drinking all the water, sending the whitefellas up the tree for bark. She was taking the piss a little bit, but it was all part of the fun.

I was really fond of a little girl called June who was a frequent flyer in the paediatric ward. She was a chubby little thing, especially considering how sick she was, and she preferred being carried around to staying in her cot. It bugged me that she kept coming back over and over again. I was curious to know why, but June was from one of the remote communities and I had no idea what was happening out there. The only people who visited these patients at home were remote area nurses, which was a whole different kind of healthcare. Remote area nurses were embedded within a community, usually in the middle of nowhere. Alice Springs wasn't much of a town, but it was still a town.

The remote nurses I met spoke very highly of the work. They loved being on the land and being immersed in the communities, which meant taking care of people when they were well as well as when they got sick. Some of the nurses went totally wild, letting their hair mat into dreadlocks, growing food on the land, joining the Aboriginal people in cultural ceremonies. I wasn't quite ready for dreads and I wasn't much of a gardener, but I liked the idea of working closely with a community with limited resources.

The only problem was that I didn't have the right experience. Remote nurses are on their own; they have to care for adults as well as kids, so I needed to expand my skills. A year after I arrived in Alice, I asked to be transferred out of the paediatrics and into the emergency department.

Emergency was so much more intense than working with kids. We saw a lot of adults with chest pains and diabetes-related issues, pneumonias and general medical conditions that were referred via us to the other speciality wards, but we also dealt with a lot of trauma—falls, breaks and wounds. Most of it was bog-standard treatment for a hospital, but some of it felt particular to the communities that we serviced.

Very soon after I'd arrived, I was tasked with cleaning a wound on an older Aboriginal woman who had come in, and given tweezers and peroxide for the job. I was expecting swabs and iodine. 'What's this?' I asked.

'It's for the maggots,' my colleague grinned. We used the peroxide to flush out the wound and the tweezers to pick out the larvae when they stuck their little heads out.'

The old lady was very relaxed and sweet, lying quietly for several hours as I flushed under the skin of her ankle and nipped at the little parasites. I developed a bit of a rhythm with it, which was good. As I would discover, there was no shortage of such patients. It didn't take long for an open wound to become flyblown in the heat, so maggots set in quickly and often in Alice Springs. I had a patient with an infected head wound further down the track, and her entire scalp was wriggling with the buggers.

The other problem that seemed particular to Alice was the road trauma. The Fink Motorcycle Race was held out there once a year and a few bike accidents always came along with it. Motorcyclists would come off at high speed on those long desert highways, and a bike collided with a camel on at least one occasion. The backpackers gave us trouble, too. We had a lot of backpackers coming through Alice Springs on their way north to south through the Red Centre, driving beaten-up Kombi vans with frayed old seatbelts. Single-vehicle accidents with seven or eight victims were pretty grim, as I discovered. We had one accident where the gas bottle in the van had come loose during the crash and crushed a young woman's chest. When they brought her in, you could see the shape of the gas bottle in her shattered rib cage.

The other category of trauma in Alice was alcohol-fuelled violence. Alcoholism was a massive problem in town and a lot of violence kicked off because people were drinking, sending reams of bloodied patients through our doors. It was a deep, long-term issue with no easy solution and it was almost mundane after a while. Just once, it was actually kind of funny.

I was manning the front desk on a particularly bad day, while the senior staff dealt with two Code 1 emergencies, a car accident and a heart attack. The department was chaotic and the waiting room was stuffed with people. Meanwhile, I was responsible for triage, which wasn't really my forte. That night, it meant dealing with a lot of short-tempered people who were sick of waiting around. In the middle of all of this, Johnny wandered in, one of the Aboriginal guys who drank in the dry riverbed that ran through the centre of town. Johnny looked like he needed a wash and he didn't smell great, and on this particular occasion he wasn't wearing shoes. A gasp rippled through the waiting room as he wandered up to the desk. *You racist bastards*, I thought. Johnny might have been a little grimy, but he was a local. I knew him well.

'Sista,' he said, 'my feet are no good.'

'What do you mean, Johnny?'

'I walked in from that town camp, all this way, and now my feet are no good.'

I looked over the counter at his bare feet and saw the skin cracked and peeling around the edges. 'Mate, we're really busy tonight,' I told him. 'I don't know if we'll be able to look at your feet.'

'Sista, they're really no good,' he insisted.

'Alright, Johnny, grab a seat. I'll see what I can do.'

As he turned away from me, I saw a huge knife wedged right between his shoulderblades. 'Jesus! Come back here,' I shouted, scrambling over the desk in my hurry to get to him. 'What happened to your back, mate?' *How are you even standing?*

Johnny peered over his own shoulder to try to get a look at the knife, like he'd just remembered it was there. 'Oh yeah,' he said. 'That no-good woman, she stab me in the back and then I have to walk all that way here from the town camp ... and now me bloody feet are no good.'

I spent eighteen months in Alice altogether: a year in paediatrics and another six months in emergency. It was a long time ago now, but working with the Aboriginal community made a huge impression on me. For all their problems, it was easy to see how deeply the community connected with the environment, and it was incredibly sad to see how disenfranchised they were, living in the town camps and settlements. But what could you do? The community was torn between their traditional way of life and the conveniences of the city. They wanted KFC and Kmart as much as anyone else, and if they wanted their kids to get an education, they had to live close to a school. They weren't nomads anymore but they weren't suburbanites either; they were stuck in this halfway place that didn't feel like home.

The health workers in Alice were pragmatic. They were motivated by problems, not overwhelmed by them. They dealt with things step-by-step, with limited resources, in the most practical way possible with a resilience you don't find in the machinery of a big city hospital. They were committed, too. Most of them still work in Aboriginal health.

I found the people who worked out there really inspiring. I didn't know exactly where I was headed when I left Alice Springs and I wanted to do some travelling. Who knew what was coming next? But wherever it was that I ended up, I knew what kind of nurse I wanted to be.

# 2

# GUERRILLAS IN THE MIST

I went to Africa when I left Alice Springs, on the rough-and-ready version of a Contiki tour. I paid $1500 to travel across the continent in the back of a four-wheel drive truck for twelve weeks, camping each night in a national park or bedding down in a backpackers' hostel. Each day, our tour group would go to the market and shop for food. At night, we'd each take turns making the group dinner. It was my first overseas trip, the first A on my list: Africa, Antarctica and the Amazon. I wanted to see the places that were changing most rapidly while I was still young enough to manage the journey. I could see Europe when I was old, I figured. Africa on a truck took stamina.

My journey began in Kenya, looping up through the Rift Valley to Uganda and down through Tanzania. We ate in iron shacks with mud floors in the middle of African slums and visited villages on the edge of vast plains, riding the bumpy roads in old bus seats bolted to the truck floor. The truck walls were made of canvas, which we rolled up on sunny days so we could watch the world go by. There were no iPhones then; no distractions. No two places felt the same.

About eight weeks before I arrived in Africa some tourists had been shot and killed in Uganda while trekking up the mountains to see the gorillas. The national park was closed, so a lot of people had cancelled their trip to that area. There were only six of us on the truck, and we were the first group after the shooting to return to the site. We set out the day after the park reopened, with an armed security escort, following the new safety protocols.

I was an enthusiastic amateur photographer—I'd done a photography course in Alice Springs—and I made the hike up into the jungle weighed down with analogue photography gear, hoping to get that perfect shot of big apes in the wild. I wasn't disappointed. At the top of the mountain we found a troop of gorillas, including two silverbacks eyeing each other off. It was really unusual to see two dominant male gorillas in one troop, but the son had just overthrown the father as leader and the old man was still lingering around.

I watched both animals through my hefty telephoto lens, shooting *click click click* through a red lens filter, which heightened the contrast of my black-and-white film. Through the viewfinder, the filter turned the apes and the jungle around them a mono-chromatic red. As I snapped photos I saw a man with a machine gun step out of the jungle, three other men appearing quickly behind him.

For a split second, I thought we were in trouble—*people died here*—but the gunmen made their way towards us calmly and our guards didn't flinch. The men I'd seen in the distance were on patrol for poachers, too, part of the security contingent that was meant to keep us safe. They didn't seem aggressive and our guards weren't tense; on reflection, their body language told me every-thing I needed to know.

I would think of that moment in years to come, when I returned to Africa. It was an interesting lesson in risk assessment. Just because someone is holding an AK-47 doesn't necessarily mean you should worry. On the other hand, as I would learn much later, being surrounded by guards with guns doesn't mean you can relax.

Later on the truck tour, we visited a Maasai Mara village in Tanzania. The villagers ran to their huts when they saw us coming, kicking off their Nikes and replacing their regular clothes with traditional woven blankets. They gathered around us, leading us from hut to hut and showing us their community, and as we walked I noticed a young girl with an ear full of pus. I was travelling with antibiotic eardrops—always carrying a first-aid kit— so it was easy to treat her. I cleaned her up and gave the drops to the girl's mother, explaining how to use them. The family was so grateful they gave me a ceremonial spear.

Ironically, those villagers and most of the others I encountered in Africa were in much better health than the people I had cared for in Alice Springs. They lived in mud huts with mud floors, but they had fewer skin and bowel infections, no scabies or runny noses. The children had clear eyes and shiny hair; they were nowhere near as malnourished as the kids in Alice.

I paid closer attention. I began to notice mothers by the side of the road, scrubbing their children in makeshift baths made from plastic buckets; mothers combing their children's hair, no matter how matted it was. The level of care those mothers took made a huge difference to the wellbeing of their children. It was health-care that started in the community, not in a hospital or clinic, and it gave me some insight into what we were missing at home.

# 3

# THE BEIRUT OF THE CAPE

When we were kids, my sister and I would each get a brand-new outfit for Christmas. On Boxing Day, we'd put on our new clothes and board a plane for Queensland. We'd fly from Sydney to Cairns in a Boeing jet and spend the night with our aunt. The next day, she'd load us onto a little twin prop and we'd fly three hours further north to see Dad.

After he and Mum separated, Dad relocated to the northernmost point of Australia, to a town called Bamaga on the tip of Cape York. It was on the edge of nowhere, in Australia's largest unspoilt wilderness. You couldn't reach it by car six months of the year because the roads flooded in the wet season.

Before we flew up to spend the holidays with Dad the first time, Mum tried to prepare us for what we would find. Bamaga was home to just a few hundred people and most of them were Aboriginal. We were little and the neighbourhood where we grew up in Sydney was blindingly white, and Mum didn't want us saying something rude because we'd been taken by surprise. She emphasised that there were a lot of Aboriginal people in Bamaga because she wanted us to be respectful, but it really backfired. My sister couldn't think of anything else. 'Look at all the black people!' she hollered, the minute we stepped off the plane. Dad had to rush over in a cloud of dust to save us from ourselves.

When I got back from Africa, I got the remote nursing job I was after, which happened to be in the same part of the world as where I'd spent summers with Dad. It was in an Aboriginal community on the west side of Cape York, in a place called Aurukun. For a tiny community, Aurukun was quite well known. It was for all the wrong reasons, unfortunately.

Aurukun had a difficult history. The first recorded contact between Europeans and Aboriginal people happened nearby, but the town itself didn't appear until the early twentieth century. It was established in 1904 as a Presbyterian mission, a government-sanctioned outpost run by religious zealots, where the people of five different Aboriginal tribes were made to live together. These tribes, collectively known as the Wik people, had been forced off their tribal lands and relocated to Aurukun, where for forty years they lived under the governance of a missionary named William MacKenzie. MacKenzie was legendary: a legendary monster. He treated the Aboriginal community as less than human, controlling people with fear and abuse, and he created the Wik people's Stolen Generation, separating children from their parents. All of this was done in the name of God's love, but the trauma it caused would resonate for generations to come. Decades after MacKenzie died, people in the community still talked about him. Almost nothing that they said about him was good.

Somewhere in this grim colonial history, alcohol was thrown into the mix, and with alcohol came violence. Aurukun developed a terrible reputation, helped along by some damning national news coverage, and by the late nineties it was considered one of the most troubled communities in Australia.

I didn't know any of this when I accepted the job, but my father did. He had resettled in Cairns by then, and was surprised when I told him the news. He said that Aurukun was known as the Beirut of the Cape, but that was all. He didn't say *don't go*, which tells you a lot about my dad. He was very laid-back. When we were kids, he took us swimming in the Jardine River, which was notoriously full of crocodiles. When I asked him about it years later, he said, 'Fewer crocs back then.'

My dad's barometer for risk was probably a little off, but it suited me. I thought his life was interesting. I'd loved those summers in Bamaga, bouncing around in the back of Dad's truck; camping and fishing, swimming with crocs.

Aurukun would be similar to Bamaga, I imagined. Being twelve hours' drive from the nearest city didn't faze me. Besides, it was meant to be a short placement. It was only when the clinic in Aurukun learned that my partner was a nurse, and that we were looking for permanent jobs, that we were both offered long-term contracts.

In hindsight, we stayed in Aurukun much longer than we should have.

In 2000, Aurukun had a school, a police station, a general store and a health clinic. The town was built at the mouth of the three major rivers: the Ward, the Watson and the Archer, which all flowed down from different parts of Cape York and met in the Gulf of Carpentaria. From the air, Aurukun was a dry little dot in a blanket of green wetlands, roughly five streets by five streets beside a red bauxite airstrip. Next to the airstrip was nothing but a tin shed and a petrol tanker. The heat was intense but it was no worse than Alice, and everywhere you looked there were trees.

On the main street, there were mango trees, planted in the early days of the mission. The old ladies in town told me that Mr MacKenzie used to make them polish the leaves, and that he whipped children who stole the fruit with the dried tail of a stingray. In another street, a long row of Queenslander houses was raised up on stilts and painted bright yellow, orange and blue. Everywhere else, the houses were made of besser block, grimy white against the red dirt roads.

Down by the boat ramp on McKenzie Drive was the one pub in town, the Three Rivers Tavern. It stood out like a sore thumb in Aurukun, the only million-dollar building in sight. Business was good. I heard the council paid the building loan off in under a year. At the time, they thought having a pub in town was better than having an alcohol ban—it was meant to stop a black market trade that was totally out of control. People would go to a lot of effort to bring booze in if the town was completely dry, but if the pub was open a few days a week, it was much harder for a smuggler to get motivated.

The Three Rivers Tavern was only open Thursday to Saturday, and only for three hours a day. It sold mid-strength beer, no take-aways, and if trouble was brewing the council would pull the shutters down. It was meant to curb demand, but it looked very much like a failure from that perspective. When I arrived in Aurukun, demand was off the charts. If trouble wasn't brewing in town, it had already boiled over.

I had my first taste of chaos the weekend after I arrived. On Friday afternoon, a car pulled up outside the clinic and a crowd of people fell out of it, screaming, carrying an unconscious man in to us. He had a swollen tongue and blocked airway, courtesy of a taipan snake—if we didn't get him breathing he would die. I was working on getting his airway open when another young guy came wandering through the front door, with a moon-shaped laceration running down the side of his face. The other nurses took care of the snakebite patient while I took a closer look at the wound. The man told me he'd been struck in the head with a stingray barb, one of the preferred weapons in town. (My colleagues told me to keep an eye on the medical supplies—young men stole bandages from the clinic to bind the spikes to their hand, then fought like skinny gladiators.) My patient now had a gaping hole in his cheek; the cut had gone clean through the flesh.

The head matron of the Aurukun Primary Healthcare Clinic was a man named Peter. He had been in Aurukun for more than six years and he had a very cool head in a crisis. Peter asked me to stitch up the facial wound but I baulked—I'd barely done any suturing in the past, and certainly not on someone's face. 'No worries, you'll be fine,' Peter said, pulling out a marker. He drew crosses on the patient's cheek so I'd know where to stitch.

I was overly cautious about washing and sterilising myself for the job, carefully slipping on surgical gloves. I still didn't feel great about doing the stitches, so I built up to it slowly. In fact, I had only just started sewing when Pete popped in to let me know the rest of the staff were escorting the snakebite victim to the airstrip. The Royal Flying Doctor Service had been called in and the patient was being evacuated. 'Sit tight,' Peter told me. 'We'll be back soon.'

There were other patients in the clinic but they were all under control, or so I was told, so I battled on with the stitches. My patient was calm as anything. He had a very high tolerance for pain, which was good, because the job was taking much longer than it should have.

Before I was done, I heard a strange noise coming from another room, a struggle, a strangled noise and a heavy thump. I walked out to see a female patient hanging from a curtain rail by a bedsheet. I had never seen anyone hang themself before and it took me by surprise. I stood there with both gloved hands in the air thinking, *Shit, I can't touch her, I'm sterile.* A second later, I snapped into action. I managed to get a shoulder underneath the woman and lifted her just enough so that I could untie the knot in the bedsheet and flop her on the bed. She fell with a thump and I winced; I'd forgotten to protect her neck. *Thank god I was strong enough to get her down by myself,* I thought, but I was really confused. I had no idea why the woman would try to kill herself.

With time, I learned that suicide attempts were common in Aurukun—a reaction to grief, sometimes a cry for help. My patient was desperate but she was lucky. As I came to learn, many attempts were successful.

I stayed with the woman until the other nurses came back, forgetting completely about the half-finished stitches and the guy with a hole in his face. By the time I returned to his room, he had disappeared. *Jesus,* I thought, *That's not good.*

Peter told me not to worry about it, that the guy would come back eventually, but a few days passed and my patient never showed, so I decided the responsible thing to do was to go out and look for him. I took another nurse from the clinic who had been in Aurukun for a while. The town wasn't particularly big and everyone knew everyone, so my colleague knew where to go.

When we pulled up at the guy's house he was sitting outside, a dark stain clearly visible across the side of his face. *Oh fuck, it's necrotic,* I thought. *I've ruined his face forever.* My colleague called the guy over and as he approached the car, I saw my needle dangling from his cheek at the end of the silk thread, and the stain spreading over the wound like black mould. It wasn't necrotic after all.

'What have you done to your face, mate?' I asked.

'The flies were bothering me,' he shrugged. 'So I covered it in Vegemite.'

Back at the clinic, I wiped the Vegemite off his face and took the stitches out, and by some miracle, the wound was fine. Not even a scar! I had survived my first week in Aurukun and no one was permanently disfigured. Not because of me, anyway.

My partner and I lived right by the airstrip, across from the police station, about fifty metres away from the morgue. We had a German Shepherd Rottweiler cross named Keita, trained to within an inch of her life. The camp dogs that roamed Aurukun weren't nearly as nice. They were always trying to bite the backs of our legs.

Aurukun was a simple community: no cinema, no shopping strip. There was a store, but it was pretty scant, and nothing resembling a restaurant. Many months after we arrived, a takeaway chicken shop opened, which was a very happy day for the community. Roast chicken with hot chips was the gourmet event of the century.

Once a month, we'd fax a grocery order to the Woolworths supermarket in Cairns, which was picked and packed and sent up to Aurukun by boat around the tip of the Cape. The vegetables were always ten days old by the time they arrived and fresh milk was impossible, but we worked out a deal with a video store in Cairns to get VHS rentals with our groceries.

On our days off, or in the afternoons when we weren't on call, we marched up and down the airstrip for exercise, watched movies or played videogames. When the weather was good, we went camping and exploring, but mostly we just worked. The clinic was slammed most of the time and there were only five health workers. We each worked up to eighty hours a week.

There were no doctors stationed in Aurukun, so the nurses were responsible for primary healthcare for the whole community. We ran vaccination programs and kept track of people with chronic conditions like diabetes or high blood pressure, and we were frontline for all the emergencies and trauma that happened in the town. Every Tuesday, a doctor flew up to run a general clinic for three days, but the rest of the time we were on our own, for better or worse. If a case was serious, we called in the Flying Doctors and patients were evacuated to Cairns.

These circumstances meant we had to do things that were otherwise unusual in nursing. The facial suture incident was just the beginning—a doctor would have done that in the city. Twice I had to intubate patients, and once I had to put a one-way valve in a man's chest to release the air pressure created by a stab wound—thankfully, by the time that happened, I'd seen the Flying Doctors perform the procedure many times. There were a lot of stabbings in town.

One night I was called in for duty along with the rest of the nursing staff because a young girl had been stabbed in the stomach, a wound about fifteen centimetres across. She had coughed and her stomach and intestines had herniated, popping out of the wound. Her organs were exposed, outside of her body, but held in place by the clear film (the periosteum) that lies under the muscles. When I arrived, she was on her side on the table with her guts hanging out of her stomach, with another massive stab wound in her back. We had to contain the herniated organs and keep them moist using cold compresses and Glad Wrap. The wound in her back was plugged with a seaweed dressing called Kaltostat, which swelled to filled the hole and stop the bleeding. In the city, even in Alice Springs, she would have been rushed into surgery, but here we had to keep her stable for a couple of hours until the Flying Doctors Service arrived.

Short of doing a medical degree, there was no better way for me to gain advanced clinical skills. I was thrown into the deep end in Aurukun and I had to learn to triage and treat critical patients, to think things through and to adapt quickly to a difficult and rapidly changing environment. It's one of the reasons I really liked Aurukun—it was an interesting place to be a nurse.

I also loved working with the community. Primary health-care had a much broader meaning in Aurukun than it had had in Alice Springs, and community service was a big part of the job. People didn't always come into the clinic when they needed to, so we went out to collect them. We treated some of the elders at home, and vaccinated some of the kids outside of town; we even took on veterinary duties now and then. (My stitches improved massively once I'd practised on a few hunting dogs. Unfortunately, my bovine patient didn't make it.)

There was a guy in town called George who I loved to visit, a lovely old bloke, skinny as anything, who wore an enormous Akubra hat. He'd been a ringer back in the day when Aurukun had its own cattle station, but the poor guy had renal tuberculosis now. We were giving him palliative care in his home, or what was left of it. When George had complained of feeling cold, his family had built a fire for him in his bedroom. It was a high-set house, completely made of wood, and they'd burned a hole right through the floor.

George was huddled in an armchair beside the hole when I went around to check on him one day, while his grandsons were out the front, playing music and mucking about. The old man had asked them for food but they didn't want to cook for him, so they'd told him he'd have to wait for the chicken shop to open. *Those lazy bastards*, I thought. George was in a bad way and he deserved better than this. I marched outside and gave the boys a serve for being so useless and told them to go and catch a fish, or go down to the general store. 'I'll be back this afternoon to check on George and he better have had something to eat!'

When I got back, the boys were gone, but I could smell roast chicken as I walked up the stairs. *Those dickheads waited for the takeaway shop to open.* When I got to George's room, he was still in the chair, but he had a drumstick the size of a brontosaurus leg in his hand.

'What on earth are you eating?' I asked.

'The boys shot me a brolga!' George grinned.

The boys had shot two brolgas, in fact, and one of them was still in the oven. It was so big that its spiny legs were sticking out of the oven door.

A couple of weeks later, I visited George again, but unfortunately he'd taken a turn. It looked like the end for the poor old bastard. The locum doctor prescribed enough morphine to manage his pain, but it was a merciful dose. We didn't expect George to wake up. I gave him the tablets and monitored him as his breathing slowed and moved in a Cheyne-Stokes pattern, a death rattle—long gaps between breaths then a heaving suck of air. *It won't be long*, I thought, but it was late, so I went home to bed. I asked the family to call me when there was some news.

I didn't get a call overnight, so I drove back out to George's place the next morning, expecting to find a corpse. Instead, I found George sitting up in his armchair, eating poultry. 'That medicine was good, sista,' he said. 'Could I get some more?'

The old bugger lasted another month.

The Wik people were superstitious about death. If someone died at home, the house were closed up for several months to allow the spirits to pass on, and it couldn't be reopened until a smoking ceremony had been performed. If someone died at the clinic, the locals would stay away, even if they were seriously ill. They were terrified of ghosts.

I was on call one Saturday night and expected it to be a quiet one—we had lost someone at the clinic the night before—but a horde of people turned up on our doorstep, huddled around a sick baby. The parents were too scared to come alone, so thirty or forty family members had come with them.

The baby needed oxygen but she was stable, which was just as well. I couldn't work with all the kids running around under my feet. The smaller ones were chasing each other between the waiting room and the trauma room, banging swinging doors as they raced in either direction. I was just about ready to crack it at them when I heard the kids stop dead in the hallway outside. Then one of the little girls started screaming.

'Right, what's going on?' I shouted, bursting out of the room.

'The dead man! The dead man went there!' They pointed. They told me they'd seen a ghost walking down the hallway and into the bathroom. I laughed and told them not to be so silly.

On Monday morning when I came into the clinic, I asked about the man who had died. He had presented late on Friday night, looking okay, but there was quite a lot of blood on his neck where he'd been stabbed. The nurse on duty had assumed that because he was walking and talking, the wound was minor, and she'd sent him to the bathroom to have a shower and clean himself up. In the shower the clot on his neck had washed away, and the man had bled out and died.

I wasn't entirely sure what to make of it. If everyone who died in Aurukun left a ghost behind, there'd be quite a few of them floating through town. There were eight murders in the three years I was there, which was astronomical for a population of under 1000 people. Most of them were the result of domestic violence. The men fought but it was the women who were killed.

Boredom was a huge part of the problem, I think. It was a town in the middle of nowhere with one shitty TV station. People had nothing to do but fish and hunt, so alcohol was a constant temptation, and the violence bubbled out of that. There were intergenerational patterns of violence, grudges handed down from father to son, stemming back to when the five separate clans were forced into close proximity. The circle of trauma went around and around, in part because there was nothing else to do.

Those who drank, drank like they were dying of thirst, or as if their alcohol would somehow disappear. It seemed partly like a hangover from a nomadic way of life where storage was a foreign concept, but there was also less likelihood that the beer would get stolen if you finished it all in one go. So many of the fights erupted over the last can of beer.

When the violence kicked off over the weekend, it was loud. Certain houses were always at the centre of the action. Music blared out of big boom boxes, people shouted in Wik language in the streets, and all the noise bled together until it sounded like a war zone. Inside the clinic, at least when I was in Aurukun, the nurses were untouchable. The community respected us and I always felt safe. But outside the clinic doors, everyone was vulnerable, especially women and children. I saw a grandmother beaten so badly that she had brain damage, because she wouldn't give her grandson the keys to the car.

The pattern was so obvious it was tragic. From Thursday to Sunday, a knot of repeat offenders would go to the pub and get smashed, and the rest of Aurukun would batten down the hatches. As long as the pub was open, there was no respite, not even on Christmas Day.

I had had steaks flown up for our first Christmas in town but my partner was called into the clinic before we could sit down to eat. I was called in shortly afterwards, steaks left cooling on the bench. The police had found a young girl who had gone missing a few days earlier. She'd been locked in a room at her boyfriend's mother's place, beaten, starving and dehydrated. The mother had colluded with her son to keep the girl hidden because he was on parole. She didn't want her son to go back to jail.

When I arrived at the clinic I found several police officers there along with the nursing staff, and everybody was pale. The minute I saw the girl, I understood why. She was mutilated, swollen black and blue, with cracked ribs and a broken jaw. Barely conscious. You got really weary of seeing people in that condition.

As we set to work trying to stabilise the patient, tensions kicked off in town, flaring up between the girl's family and the boyfriend's clan. That was part of the pattern too, escalating violence. Sometimes it would last the whole weekend. That day, we had a trail of patients falling through the clinic doors and we didn't get back to the house until 2 a.m. Christmas was over by then. There was no point in celebrating. And anyway, our Rottweiler had eaten the steaks.

As hard as it might have been for the nursing team in Aurukun, the police had it worse. There were five officers in town, facing constant threats. They were first on the scene whenever violence was brewing and it was their job to get in the way, to try to settle things down. They were an easy target if people were angry, and more than once they had to lock themselves in the station while people rioted outside. At least one of the officers I worked with in Aurukun experienced serious PTSD. They just never knew which way things were going to go, and that constant tension was damaging. I felt like I was immune to the stress in the clinic, but I had a lot of sympathy for those cops.

One evening, when the town was seriously divided and it seemed like all hell was about to break loose, one of the officers called and asked me to bring the old F100 ambulance out to help settle the situation. We only used that ambulance to transport dead bodies, so the townspeople were terrified of it.

I went down with lights and sirens blaring, and parked in between two rival mobs that were ready to go off at each other. They were holding rocks and sticks, and shouting in language from opposite sides of the street. The officer who had called me was speaking to elders from each side of the conflict, trying to calm things down, but things were clearly too far gone to avoid a full-on brawl.

'We can't hold this back,' I reasoned. 'Can we not just take the weapons off them?'

We told the elders that the two mobs could fight, but only with their fists, and the officers and I walked through the crowd, taking bricks and bars out of people's hands, and piling them up beside the ambulance. When we were done, we took a seat on the bonnet of the car and waited for things to kick off. Right in front of us, eighty or so people from town starting laying into each other, a mess of shouting and flailing limbs. I'd never seen anything like it. One by one, the men dropped out of the fight and came to sit beside the ambulance, so I pulled out the first-aid kit. One by one, in the order they arrived, I patched them up and sent them home.

At some point, I decided that the old women in town needed a break from the weekend chaos, so I started up a little picnic club. I picked them up on a Friday afternoon and drove them down to the boat ramp, setting them up with lemonade and chips. They sat on camp chairs or blankets, weaving and fishing, until I drove back and took them all home to bed.

One week, we were particularly busy in the clinic so I didn't manage to get back to collect my charges until after sunset. When I arrived, my headlights swung over an empty riverbank and I nearly had a heart attack. The ladies had climbed down into the water to gather baitfish, but they weren't alone. I saw a big, dark shadow and red reptilian eyes out in the river. We didn't swim in Aurukun, and for a very good reason. 'Get out! Get out of the water!' I shouted, running to the edge. 'What on earth are you doing?'

One of the women was an amputee, so she was very slow to respond. 'Don't think about it, sista,' she called, as she hopped and swam to shore. 'You know, if you don't think about the crocodiles, they don't think about you.'

There was a small group of kids in Aurukun that was increasingly involved in petrol sniffing. The kids were bored, just like the adults, and it was a cheap and dirty form of entertainment. It was poison, too, and the effects could be absolutely devastating. We started to see the kids at the clinic, presenting with lung and respiratory issues. In the long term, it would mean brain damage and major organ failure. Some people saw petrol sniffing as a social issue, but it was a health problem, as far as I was concerned. I just had to think creatively about how to treat it.

I met with a couple of kids who were attending school regularly to brainstorm a solution, and one of them mentioned the abandoned radio station in town. There were a few places like that in Aurukun, which had opened with a burst of government funding and fallen into disuse when the funds had dried up. The radio station was simple enough, just two rooms in a besser-block building, but all the gear was still ready and waiting for a little community radio show.

I decided to run with the Rock Eisteddfod model, a performing arts program I remembered from school that was 100 per cent drug- and alcohol-free. We would form a little club to launch the Three Rivers youth radio station, but anyone who wanted to get involved had to stay at school and stay away from petrol.

I was the supervisor, but the kids ran the show. They came up with the name 3-Ray and a little sun logo, which we had printed on T-shirts down in Cairns. They sold a few in town to raise money to buy CDs. Once a week, in a two-hour broadcast, they would chat and play music, make up funny skits and shout out to friends who were listening. In between their banter and the music, I snuck in a few health messages. We made up adverts about nutrition and hygiene, including songs and jingles that the kids would perform on air. They worked on them during the week and brought them into the show, which was my strategy for keeping the kids busy when I wasn't around.

3-Ray was quite a hit in the community. The kids wore their T-shirts proudly and their elders listened to the show, and it became a real badge of achievement for anyone involved. It wasn't a magic bullet, but it was certainly helping to keep the kids occupied. I decided to expand the project into a blue-light disco—a safe space for kids under twelve that was drug- and alcohol-free, just like the radio station. Once a month, I connected a sound system to some speakers in an old canteen building in town, and the kids would come along with their chaperones to dance and muck about. The day before each dance, I would drive around town and remind them—no petrol. If I could smell it on them when they arrived, the kids didn't get in. The disco was only one day a month, so it couldn't make a massive difference, but it was something. Something was better than nothing, I figured. It was the best I could do.

The greatest thing about the blue-light disco was that the parents and grandparents got involved, laughing and dancing with the kids. Towards the end of the project, there were 150 people coming along every time we held the event. It was something I organised alone, when I wasn't rostered at the clinic, and it was almost more than I could handle, but it was worth it. The discos were held on Wednesdays, so the pub was closed, and everyone was in a good mood. A peaceful night out in Aurukun was a welcome change of pace.

When the pub was closed in Aurukun, kids would play cricket in the street, families would go fishing together. Sometimes, we would go to see concerts at the school, where the kids sang traditional songs and did tribal dances, still very much a part of their culture. There were many beautiful people in Aurukun who I respected, but they weren't the ones who consumed most of my attention. As a nurse, I had a biased perspective, and it was usually focused on what was going wrong. Over time, it wasn't the peaceful part of the community that left the biggest impression. It was the alcoholism that rolled in over the weekend and the violence that never seemed to stop. It wore me down.

The last birthday I celebrated in Aurukun was the worst I've ever had. I was having a party with the team from the clinic, along with some schoolteachers and police officers from town, and everyone except the nurse on call had had a drink or two. The phone rang and the nurse was called in. It rang again, and a second nurse followed. It rang for the third time, which was never a good sign, and a third nurse headed into the clinic.

After two off-duty police officers had been called away from the party, the phone rang once more for my partner and me. The police had a major case in a house right across the road from ours and they needed more help—it was serious. We'd both been drinking, but what choice did we have? We were the only two nurses left.

Across the road, we were led around police tape and into the house. It was completely empty except for a tricycle and a woman sleeping in the hallway. The rooms were bare and the walls were covered in grime. Someone called out to us from the back of the house and we ran towards them, right into the scene of a nightmare. In the back room, we found a woman on the ground who looked as though her head had been cut off. The whole room was covered in blood. Somehow, she was still alive. She was breathing through the wound in her neck.

We knew this woman. She'd been a victim of domestic violence before and her husband had been sent to jail. When the men went to jail, they had decent food, no alcohol and a gym. They came back bigger, stronger and much more dangerous than before.

I wanted to intubate the woman, but that was a crazy idea. We wouldn't have been able to manage the severed carotid artery; we didn't have any blood in the clinic. My partner told me to go to the clinic and prep the trauma room, trying to distract me. We both knew that the woman wasn't going to make it.

Back in the clinic, I got the call to switch on the refrigerated room we used as a morgue. The woman in the house had died and they were bringing her body over. The morgue wasn't always in use; we only turned it on when somebody died.

Once I'd flipped the switch, there was nothing else for me to do. I walked back to our house, the woman's blood all over my clothes. At home, the party was still going. The remaining guests were teachers, not nurses or emergency workers, so I couldn't tell them what had happened. I couldn't and I wouldn't. I didn't want to talk about it, I just wanted to get back to the party. I went to the bathroom to clean myself up and joined my friends without mentioning a thing. It didn't occur to me for a second that my behaviour was unusual. It was just another night in Aurukun.

I was drunk and laughing when my partner finally came home, horrified to find the party in full swing. My partner did what I probably should have done, clearing everyone out of the house. We fought, but my arguments sounded weak. *It wasn't my shift. I did what I could. It's my birthday.* But how could I have seen what I saw that night, then walked home and cracked open a merry beer? *You're overreacting. If I fell into a heap every time I saw something horrible here, I wouldn't be able to function.*

It took a long time for me to see that my partner was right. As months turned into years, all the violence and trauma in Aurukun had become normal to me. I felt numb to it, but that in itself was a problem, and the fact that I wasn't alone probably made it worse. One night, I was at a party at someone else's place, one of the other nurses. We saw the ambulance pull up outside the morgue, which meant that someone in the community had died. We all knew the most likely victims. We took bets on who it was.

Bleak humour was very useful in Aurukun. We did the absolute best we could to serve the community but we were there to stitch up the wounds. We couldn't stop them from happening. After a while, you had to laugh, just to break the tension. But I got to the point where I couldn't make jokes and I really couldn't take it anymore.

It was the kids, in the end. We found twenty kids in the community infected with syphilis. The oldest was seventeen and the youngest was three. We thought it had been transmitted between children that were seven or eight years old, through simulated sex. They shared rooms with the parents and were exposed to sexual intercourse at a very young age. It was common for young children in the community to mimic what they saw. Some of the disease was transmitted through consensual sex between teenagers, but that's not where it started. At some point the disease had been introduced by an adult in the community.

I did a lot of work with the kids to establish the chain of transmission. I used every ounce of trust and influence that I had built with them in at the radio station and the blue-light disco to figure out how it had happened. And then I reported it, as I had to, to Queensland social services.

After all of that, only one person was charged, a seventeen-year-old boy. He had had consensual sex with a fourteen-year-old who was openly gay and was charged with carnal knowledge of a minor. I suspected that the younger kid, the fourteen-year-old, had been a victim of incest and I had written as much in my report, but it was never properly investigated because the community wouldn't allow it. The two gay kids were targeted and the rest of the kids were left vulnerable to abuse, and on top of everything else I had managed to break their trust. And that broke my spirit. I think I'd just had enough.

Like the people in town, the nurses who stayed too long in Aurukun drank too much. The stress was a quiet rot. In the three years I had been there, I had put on a lot of weight, and towards the end I was angry all the time. I was eight weeks shy of a $6000 bonus when I decided to leave. The other nurses thought I was mad not to wait it out, but I didn't care about the money. I felt like I might not leave at all if I didn't get out immediately, and something inside of me knew it was time to go.

My partner and I separated and I went back to Brisbane, where I had bought a house. I spent the next three months doing nothing, decompressing. Aurukun was the toughest place I would ever work, worse than anything to come, but there was no formal debriefing process when you worked up there. I had to figure out how to take care of myself. Every morning, for three months, I went for a swim. Every afternoon, I painted my house. I couldn't stand hearing people's opinions about all the troubles in Aurukun so I avoided talking about it. In fact, for the better part of three months, I didn't talk much at all. I actually didn't realise that I was in a bad way, not at the time. I just wanted to be alone for a while.

# 4

# LOVE YOUR COWS,
# JUST DON'T 'LOVE' YOUR COWS

In 1859, a Swiss businessman named Henry Dunant witnessed a bloody clash between France and Austria that left 40,000 men dead or wounded on the battlefield. Shocked by the carnage, and the total lack of medical care for the soldiers, Dunant convinced the local population to help nurse the wounded. The soldiers received treatment no matter which side they fought on and their nurses, women from the surrounding villages, were neutral in the battle. Later, Dunant wrote a book about his experiences, advocating for national volunteer organisations to preserve the dignity of soldiers in war. This was the birth of the Red Cross, one of the oldest and most recognised humanitarian organisations in the world.

Today, the Red Cross is a vast network of national societies, each funded by their own national government and supported by a governing body, the International Federation of the Red Cross (IFRC). Together with the International Committee of the Red Cross (ICRC), which is responsible for field operations in conflict settings, the national societies look after victims of war and disaster. They are also involved in development work in areas of conflict, crisis and poverty. And everywhere, on every mission, they remain neutral and independent.

I didn't know much about the organisation when I applied to join it in 2003. For anyone looking to get into humanitarian aid, working for the Red Cross was a dream role, a chance to be deployed into conflict and disaster zones around the world. I hadn't really thought about doing humanitarian work, but I missed the challenge of working remotely. I'd spent nine months as a high school nurse in Brisbane and I was really over it. I wanted to go out into the world and get my hands dirty again.

I was interviewed by the field personnel manager for the Australian Red Cross, a woman named Charlotte, who recruited local nurses for international missions with the ICRC. Charlotte was particularly interested in my work in Cape York. She had completed Red Cross missions around the world, in many a disaster and conflict zone, but she hadn't survived more than a few weeks of nursing in Aurukun. 'How did you do three years?' she asked.

'I dunno, I thought it was really fun,' I shrugged. The work had been challenging and I liked living in that part of the world. The trauma had subsided by then. It was an honest answer. It also turned out to be the right one.

My qualifications weren't up to scratch and my résumé was a disaster, but those were fixable problems, as far as Charlotte was concerned. She made me enrol in a Master of Public Health degree and helped me to rewrite my résumé before she sent it up the chain, because she'd decided that I had the right stuff for the Red Cross. You couldn't buy the experience I had had in Aurukun.

My new job began with a weeklong induction program, Red Cross training camp, where I spent a lot of time learning about

Henry Dunant and the fundamental principles of the organisation. The Red Cross derives its mandate from the Geneva Conventions and takes its principles very seriously, relying on impartiality, neutrality, independence and humanity to provide aid to victims without being harmed. This stuff was drummed into us like a mantra. People who joined the Red Cross did noble, difficult work. Of course, there was no guarantee we'd be up to it.

We weren't just being trained at camp, we were being watched, and part of the process was to determine if we were suitable for the work. While we learned necessary skills like radio communications and conflict resolution, the trainers did their best to unsettle us, to evaluate how we might react under stress. After several days at the same desks, we left the room and came back to find our books had been moved around, without explanation. One night, we turned up to dinner to find there was no cutlery. These were very small things, but they were telling. Small things really bothered some people.

Towards the end of the training, the Army Reserve burst into our classroom and held us at gunpoint. They came in full camouflage gear, holding machine guns, and asked to speak to the person in charge, demanding medical personnel to come and treat injured soldiers at their base. They took two doctors and a nurse out of the room, we heard two gunshots outside, *bang bang*, and it was over.

We knew it was a drill, obviously. We knew the people who were taken out of the room weren't in any real danger, but as a drill, it was surprisingly effective. It was a shock to the system and it made our adrenalin surge, weeding out a couple of unsuitable candidates in the process. One had worked in the field previously and had PTSD following a security incident. The other guy was ex-army; too alpha. He had tried to take over control of the exercise and he'd failed the test.

In the debrief, the instructors told us we had to drill these kinds of scenarios because we needed to be able to respond effectively in real life and not be overwhelmed. Security incidents in the field were not common, but they did happen. It was no good giggling nervously because the situation seemed unreal. Laughing in a soldier's face could get you killed.

I passed basic training and joined the Red Cross roster, ready to be deployed at any moment. Nine months later, they finally had a mission for me.

The Red Cross wanted someone with two or three years' experience in international aid to run a program in South Sudan. Two nurses had taken the job, one after the other, and both had quit before the end of their contracts because they couldn't handle the living conditions. Charlotte had gone in to bat for me, convincing the ICRC that I would stay out my contract and that I would be operational very quickly, despite not having the requisite experience. To be operational in the Red Cross meant having skills that were specific to the field: being able to handle a four-wheel drive vehicle and operate a two-way radio; being comfortable with and conscious of security protocols. That kind of stuff was second nature to me already. Charlotte had faith that I would do well and she convinced the Red Cross to give me a go.

Ten days after I got the call, I was on a plane bound for Khartoum, the northern capital of Sudan. There was a lot of humanitarian aid traffic into the country because of the trouble brewing in the western region of Darfur, where a mounted Islamic militia, referred to as the Janjaweed, was active in villages. The head of water and sanitation operations in Khartoum barely had time to see me before I boarded another plane south, but he did give me one useful piece of advice. He told me to sit tight for at least three months, and do nothing. I was headed for a place called Yirol in the centre of South Sudan, to manage a hygiene promotion program that had been running for two years already. It was running very well, he said, so I shouldn't feel the need to make any changes. 'You're an expat, not an expert,' he said. 'Keep your mouth shut and your eyes open.'

From Khartoum, I flew to a town in Kenya called Lokichogio, a humanitarian hub that had sprung up during the second Sudanese civil war, which started in 1983. For twenty years, opposition forces in South Sudan had been fighting the north for independence. The only safe place for aid organisations to set up operations had been across the border in Kenya, where the Red Cross had built a hospital and a sizeable compound for its staff. From Loki, the Red Cross ran air missions in and out of South Sudan, bringing the wounded back for lifesaving surgery and treatment.

There was only one Red Cross mission running inside South Sudan, and that's where I was headed. After a short induction, I hopped a ride on the next cargo plane out of Lokichogio, headed for Yirol, a little speck in the middle of the country. There was a small group of expats there, working out of a small hospital, living in a rustic little compound. That was where I was going to spend the next twelve months of my life.

From the window of the plane, I saw rippling waves of millet fields. It looked so lush from the air, but looks could be deceiving. The rains had come and the millet had grown taller than my head, but it wasn't ready to harvest yet and food stores from the previous year had run out. As I learned later, they called it the hunger period.

Beside the vast fields of green, clustered around Yirol Lake, I saw the grass-thatched roofs of *tukuls*—Sudanese mud huts—with intricate dirt paths winding around the circular buildings. A single street made of pressed brown dirt stretched south past the Yirol marketplace towards the army barracks; a street that was lined with mango trees, just like in Aurukun. A second street ran at a right angle to the main street, past the Red Cross hospital to the staff compound. These were the only concrete buildings I could see that did not have obvious damage from the fighting.

A Colombian obstetrician called Isabella collected me from the airstrip. She was a tiny, long-haired woman, pissed off to discover that I was on my first mission. Two women before me had quit before the end of their contracts and left the team in the lurch, and Isabella didn't want another flake on her hands. She asked if I had any practical experience using a two-way radio. I told her I had been a surf lifesaver in Brisbane and I had run the control room. She asked if I minded showering outside, if I liked cooking, if I knew how to handle a four-wheel drive vehicle. She told me they had enough LandCruisers to get around but not enough drivers, so I better be happy behind the wheel and 15 centimetres deep in mud. 'Not a problem,' I told her. These were some of my favourite things.

Yirol was even smaller than Aurukun. Local people padded the streets in tattered second-hand clothes. The people were very tall, very thin and very curious, staring openly at my unfamiliar white face through the window of the LandCruiser. Children wandered around in oversized rags or nothing at all, and smiled at me through the glass. Beyond the road, there was tall grass, green shrubs and spindly acacia trees.

Isabella pointed out the hospital as we drove past. The Red Cross had chosen Yirol as its base of operations in South Sudan because the hospital was already there, built during the British colonial period in the first half of the twentieth century. With a little renovation work, it had been restored to a functioning clinic, with an in-patient ward, an out-patient ward and one for maternity care. Isabella ran the maternity ward while a French doctor named Victor ran the other two. A Swiss nurse named Audrey also worked on the team, running an onchocerciasis control program—she was trying to limit the impact of 'river blindness' on the population of South Sudan. Louis, the head of office, was also Swiss, a chef and veteran of multiple Red Cross missions. He was deeply attached to the two cats that lived in the Red Cross compound.

Finally, there was Leo, a water and sanitation engineer with whom I would be working very closely. Leo was in charge of drilling boreholes for villages across the surrounding regions and I was supposed to teach the communities how to use them properly. This is just one of the things the Red Cross would do in a war zone. Water is a lifesaving and highly valued commodity, and by committing to long-term water security projects the Red Cross was able to build trust within conflict zones. This allowed the organisation to do some of its more sensitive work, like caring for prisoners of war, providing protection to civilians and explaining the 'rules of war' to opposing military forces. Now that the civil war in Sudan was winding down, and South Sudan was on the verge of being declared an independent country, the Red Cross was making good on its water security promise. The organisation had identified a long list of sites where boreholes were necessary—eighty sites where it hoped to drill over a three-year program.

I didn't know much about water and sanitation when I arrived and there wasn't much of a briefing. What I needed to know about the program, I would learn from books that were waiting for me in Yirol. I kept my mouth shut, my eyes open and I read.

I would be responsible for hygiene promotion. Having a clean water source wasn't enough; the community needed to take ownership of it, to ensure that it would be maintained properly whether or not the Red Cross was around. *How do you keep water clean? How do you use it to clean yourself and your environment? And how does having clean water affect the health of your community?* Things that seemed obvious in Australia were not obvious in South Sudan. It was my job to start introducing these concepts.

I had a team of local staff that had been working on the program long before I arrived, who did most of the heavy lifting. With a bit of steering from me, the team would help the community to decide where their water pump should be located. The community would collect raw materials that were necessary for the project and they would make decisions about how to manage the supply. Did women from the village have to stay in line all day for water or could they leave their jerry cans in line? Could animals from the village drink from the pump? Who would clean the pump if it was dirty? There were a lot of things that had to be nutted out.

Once the drill team had come in and built the pump, we would go back and run the hygiene program, teaching the community about germs, about why they get sick, and why clean water is crucial to good health. My job was to sit under a tree and teach people to wash their hands, essentially. Not quite as sexy as I had imagined, but I really loved it.

The Sudanese people were very happy and very practical, for the most part. After twenty years of war, they had developed a deep resilience and they were very matter-of-fact about survival. When help was offered, they made the most of it, and that made my work incredibly satisfying.

By the time I arrived, all of the borehole sites closest to Yirol had been completed so I was driving up to two hours a day to reach the next villages on the list. It wasn't normal for an expat to drive the Red Cross vehicle in South Sudan, but none of the Sudanese staff had driver's licences and there was no way for them to take the test in Yirol, so I became the designated driver.

The local team would run the water and sanitation training in Dinka, the local language, while I sat by looking for non-verbal cues that things were getting off track. We were supposed to facilitate the discussion and let the community come to their own conclusions, not just give them the answers. Taking owner-ship over the process was key to their success. But obviously, we already knew what the answers should be and how we could offer support. The Red Cross team had to walk a very tricky line between facilitation and instruction to get the best outcomes for the community, which involved asking a lot of leading ques-tions and nudging the discussion along. My job was to try to stop my team from outright teaching, which was much harder than it sounds. It seemed difficult for the local staff to act like they didn't already know the answers to the questions people were asking.

The best part of my day was when we arrived in a village and sat down to wait for the community to come together. We would spread a large tarpaulin under a tree and prepare tea with sugar for our guests. Sugar was like gold in South Sudan, so it was a great enticement for people to join us, but it could still take a long while for everyone to arrive. In planting season, we could be waiting two and a half hours.

The older women would arrive first, a piece of nylon fabric tied over one shoulder and strings of bright beads around their necks, and we would chat with them to pass the time until the rest of the community turned up. The women always had questions for me and they were rarely about water. I was tall and broad, and I always wore pants. I had authority because I drove the car, and many people misunderstood 'Amanda' as 'Commander', which was the closest English word they knew, so I got a lot of questions about my gender. Straight up, 'Are you a man or a woman?'

It didn't bother me, but my Sudanese staff members could be very protective. Once, I noticed a team member called Josie stiffen because she didn't like the question a man had asked. I was worried there was some kind of security issue and insisted she repeat what she had heard. Reluctantly, Josie said, 'He wants to know if you have a vagina.'

I laughed, but the man was serious and now the whole community was staring at me. 'Yes, I do,' I told them solemnly. *Thanks for asking!*

The Sudanese people wanted to know why my arms were so hairy. Their skin was completely smooth, they had no body hair at all. The children were so curious about it that it would be a matter of minutes before one of them crawled into my lap and started stroking my arms, plucking at my arm hair. They liked to touch the hair on my head as well, which was blonde and fine and radically different to their own coarse black coils. I sometimes pulled my hair out of its ponytail and gave it a good shake, just to hear the kids squeal and run. They thought I looked like a lion.

Once the villagers accepted that I was a woman, the questions really started to flow, and always in the same direction. I was asked about marriage and children. This happened so frequently that I learned to have the conversation in Dinka. I was a white person, a *kawaaga*, so I had special status. The villagers assumed that I was wealthy, so naturally I'd make a great catch. Grandmothers in particular wanted to know if I was on the market; they would often sneak up behind me and measure my hips with their hands. *Good hips.* Wide hips meant less chance of death in childbirth, which meant I'd be a good investment.

One of my team members, a man named Kamal, became very good at negotiating my bride price. He thought it was very funny, though it was always done with a straight face, and when he was finished, I would have to talk myself out of trouble. 'I can't carry the water on my head,' I would explain to the women.

'Don't be silly, you're in charge of the water,' they would scoff. 'Just put the pump next to your house.'

'But I don't know how to pound the maize!'

'We will get you a second wife to pound the maize.'

In the end, the only really good excuse I had was that my father lived very far away. We could agree to a bride price of 400 cows, but they couldn't ship the cows to Australia. Towards the end of my time in South Sudan, a local man came to the Red Cross compound with a new offer. He had figured out the cow problem, he said. He would sell the cows and transfer the profits to my father via Western Union.

Even after they had accepted that I was a woman, the villagers struggled to understand what kind of woman I was. I didn't fit any of the moulds of Sudanese life and there was no TV or film to give them insight into other cultures of the world. They lived in mud huts and raised cattle; their primary concerns were the safety of their family, their cows and where their next meal was coming from.

One day I met two girls in their late teens, both of whom had had children, who wanted to know how long I had been at school. 'Sixteen years,' I told them. To be really educated in South Sudan at the time was to have reached fourth grade at around nine years old—the education system had all but collapsed during the war. To be really, truly educated, you studied for six or seven years, so sixteen years sounded totally ridiculous to these girls. It was almost as long as they had been alive. What could I possibly need to learn that would keep me at school for sixteen years?

Like everyone else, the girls asked if I was married.

'No.'

'Will you have children?'

'I think so, yes.'

'How many children?'

'Probably two.'

'Only two?!' they tutted.

'Children are very expensive,' I laughed.

'But you are white, you are rich,' they argued.

'I am not rich in my country. Food is very expensive,' I told them, but they struggled to understand. 'I can't grow food, I have no garden. I have to buy it in the market, it is expensive.'

'What about food that comes from the air?' they asked.

These young women had grown up during the civil war, when humanitarian aid planes had flown overhead every season and dropped sacks of maize from the sky. They assumed this was something that happened everywhere.

Moving into the Red Cross compound in Yirol was like moving into an incredibly intense share house. My teammates were excited to have someone new to talk to, some fresh blood in a very remote part of the world. In situations like this, you found commonalities, not differences, and became very close to people you might never have been friends with at home. From day one, I was cooking and eating every meal with the same five people. There were no movies to escape to, no television to watch, so getting to know each other was our best form of entertainment. I got to know way too much about Victor's love life, for example. He was very popular with the ladies in Loki.

There was a generator and solar panels in the Red Cross compound, so we had power, unlike the rest of Yirol, though it cut out in the evening. The fans would stop running just as we were heading to bed, leaving us to sweat it out in our little concrete bunkers, in 45-degree heat. The only way to survive it was to soak your bedsheet in a bucket of water and spread it over your baking skin. Within a couple of hours, the sheet would be bone-dry again.

When the power was on, it had a downside. At night, our compound was the only light source for a hundred kilometres, which made us a beacon for every bug and insect known to humankind. The bugs hung so thick in the air that the noise of their beating wings would keep me awake, so one night I decided to take matters into my own hands. I found a spray bottle and some chemicals in the storage room, donned overalls and a pair of Oakley sunglasses, and went after the bugs like the Terminator. It took our cleaners two days to sweep up the carnage.

But even with the heat and the bugs, we lived like kings, at least relative to the rest of South Sudan. Our food was shipped in from Loki and we had a mechanical water pump in the compound, which meant that we had flushing toilets. We had two showers, one for the girls and one for the boys, though admittedly they were outside. And every two weeks, just when the austerity was getting too much, we'd be flown out to Loki for a rostered weekend off, where we'd drink at one of the local bars or swim in the pool at the Trackmark Hotel.

Back in Yirol, we had to make our own fun or we didn't get any. Sometimes my teammates would spend whole evenings speaking in different languages—one night Italian, one night French, one night German. I wish I could say that I learned a few words. It sounded great, but I had no idea what anyone was saying. If I needed to tune out, I listened to one of the 350 songs I had on my first generation iPod.

In this context, getting packages from home was pretty much the greatest thing in the world. We got regular post in Yirol, but packages were strictly limited to under a kilogram, and my friends at home took this rule very seriously. They would stand at the post office in Australia adding individual Fantales or Minties to a cardboard box until they hit exactly 999 grams. For my birthday in South Sudan, I got a party in a box, with cake mix, streamers and even candles. For Australia Day, my friend sent me a blow-up kangaroo and Aussie flag tattoos, plus a tube of Vegemite and some white zinc. I couldn't have been happier.

Beyond that, there wasn't a lot of communication with the outside world. In Lokichogio, the entire Red Cross compound shared three computers and paid for internet access by the minute. In Yirol, messages came in rich text format over the radio network—I'd spend hours trying to download four messages some nights. We listened to the BBC world radio service so we heard the news, but it was less impactful somehow without the pictures. Once a week, we'd get a copy of *Time* magazine and we'd have to piece everything together. When the Indian Ocean tsunami happened on Boxing Day in 2004, for example, we heard about it but had no television coverage, so we couldn't really appreciate the scale. It wasn't until we got the next issue of *Time* that we understood how devastating it was.

When my teammates had rostered weekends in Loki, I would lend a hand in the hospital. I also stepped up if there was a health crisis, which happened every now and then. At one point, a series of patients presented with symptoms that none of us had seen before, though we had an inkling of what they might be. The patients had severe aquaphobia, or fear of water. Even the dripping IV line would trigger a response—they'd see it and become extremely agitated, to the point of having a fit, and they'd make what sounded like a growling or barking sound in the backs of their throats. We had no internet, so we discussed it among ourselves and called in to Lokichogio for a consultation. Everyone agreed the symptoms were textbook: we were looking at a rabies outbreak. The problem was that once the symptoms had presented, there was nothing we could do.

The first patient was a ten-year-old boy who had been bitten by a dog a few months earlier. He was having horrific spasms and 'barking' constantly. His family was really distressed. Only a handful of cases around the world had survived rabies once it had progressed to this stage, and all of those cases had been in tertiary hospitals with state-of-the-art intensive care units. We didn't have the facilities or staff to manage the young boy and he was suffering horribly. He was so agitated that he presented a significant risk of infection to others; he'd already bitten his uncle. There was nothing we could do but isolate him. The boy suffered, dehydrated and convulsing, on the veranda of a disused building at the back of the hospital. He died within a few days.

When two more cases came in, our worry grew. How many cases could there be? We sat down with the local military to discuss a plan. Clearly there were rabid dogs in the area, but if people were treated immediately after being bitten, rabies wouldn't develop. The fatal progression of the disease was preventable with a vaccine, if it was given in time. But the vaccine was hard to get, it was expensive and it had a complicated dosage schedule—you needed three injections up to two weeks apart. It would be challenging in this environment.

To make matters worse, the World Health Organization (WHO) only had three doses of rabies vaccine in stock locally, which were flown in the next day. One went to the uncle of the boy who had died, but the other two we kept on hand, and we spread the word that anyone who had been bitten should come in to see us. The community began to panic and people arrived, demanding treatment for dog bites sustained years earlier. We held the remaining vaccine doses back, waiting for some evidence that the disease had been transmitted, stuck between a rock and a hard place. In the meantime, the army went to work on the source. They put the word out that dogs were carrying a life-threatening disease, then for two days they travelled from hut to hut, shooting every dog on sight.

I don't think this approach would have worked anywhere else in the world. It was a logical solution but one that would not be easy for a lot of people to accept. The dogs in Yirol weren't as pampered or domesticated as the ones back home, but they weren't wild; each of them was connected to a family. Yet their owners didn't complain when they were culled, in fact they saw it as a positive thing. There were so many things that killed these people that they could not control—war, malaria, complications from childbirth—that they did everything they could to save themselves when given the chance.

If we had wanted to cull cattle, it would have been a different story. Cows were money in South Sudan because the local currency was basically worthless. South Sudanese pounds, introduced by the British, had not been printed since before the civil war. The notes that remained in circulation were almost black and falling to pieces, their value indistinguishable. Wealth was measured by the size and quality of your herd, and people kept a very close eye on their stock. Sometimes too close.

There were nomadic families around Yirol that travelled and lived with their cattle, which was a nightmare from a public health point of view. The mortality rate for children under five years old in these families was much higher than in the static communities. Malaria, pneumonia and diarrhoea were the main culprits, but a number of cultural practices put the communities at high risk for other diseases. One of them was brucellosis, known as undulating fever, a bacterial disease that causes brutal fevers, night sweats and crippling pain, and can be followed by arthritis, fatigue and even death. It is transmitted by close contact with the body fluids of infected animals.

I was sent out to investigate health conditions in the cattle camps, to figure out why their health outcomes were so poor, and as I discovered, the list of risk factors was long. These families lived with their cows—not next to, or close too, but *with* their cows, which meant they were surrounded by cow shit all day. They were covered in cow shit, quite literally, because they burned the manure and spread it on their bodies to ward off mosquitos. (I don't know if it worked, but they were convinced that it did.) They used cow urine to bleach their hair, putting their heads directly under the hot stream of piss as it erupted from the animals. They also drank unpasteurised milk; they weren't vaccinated; they didn't use mosquito nets. And of course, there was no clean water source in the nomadic camps and regular handwashing had never crossed anyone's mind.

When it came to taking care of the herd, different tasks were allocated to different age groups, and they each presented different problems. The young boys were in charge of herding the cows over long distances, putting them at high risk of guinea worm infection, but it was the task allocated to the young girls that concerned me the most. They performed something that looked sexual on the cows. It wasn't sexual, it was just part of their farming practices, but I found it pretty confronting. When cows stopped producing enough milk, the young girls in the camps would put their face inside the cows' vaginas and blow raspberries, using the vibrations to stimulate milk production. This was how the girls were getting brucellosis.

It takes time to change ingrained cultural practices like this, so we tried to think of practical solutions. Could we distribute dental dams? How about a health campaign: *Love your cows, just don't 'love' your cows!* In the end, all we could do was ask that girls come to see us for antibiotics as soon as they developed symptoms.

The cattle camps presented some unique challenges for me, but they could be very peaceful too, especially at sunset. When the temperature dropped, steam rose from the cow pats, which looked almost like mist. It made for some great photographs. The Sudanese people were incredibly photogenic, too—very statuesque and elegant, even when covered in cow shit. Their lives were harsh but in the right light, even a harsh life can look beautiful.

The complications arising from local cultural practices extended beyond the cattle camps. Most of the women in South Sudan gave birth at home and there were many beliefs and misconceptions that made their childbirth dangerous. The women believed that they couldn't drink once labour started, for example, because it would put the baby at risk of drowning. We had no luck convincing them otherwise.

It was only when the traditional birth attendants thought there may be a problem that women were referred to our maternity clinic, so the cases that Isabella and her midwives dealt with were always especially difficult. Isabella was an incredible obstetrician—she had worked in Colombia in low-resource settings before coming to South Sudan so she was highly skilled and very calm, and she took most things in her stride. If I was called in as an extra pair of hands, it usually meant things were really going sideways.

She called me back from the field urgently one day to help with a particularly bad case, so I arrived covered in mud and dust, sweating from hours out in the sun. Unfortunately, the mother Isabella was dealing with was in far worse shape. It was a breech birth and the mother was going into shock, and Isabella had her hands buried inside her, trying to get the baby out. The baby had died in utero several days earlier and now there was a risk that the mother would die, too.

The obstetrics room was built of besser blocks, with a small window covered by worn wooden shutters. It looked more like a shed than part of a hospital. There was a black chair with stirrups in the centre of the room, and a single spotlight, run by battery. Beside the chair, there was a steel table that held sterile equipment.

Lying back in the chair, the mother was completely silent. She was covered in beads of sweat, struggling to remain conscious as Isabella wrestled with her baby's corpse.

When the body emerged, it was barely recognisable. It was blueish because it was completely devoid of oxygen, but grey where the skin had started to slough away inside the womb. The legs emerged, then the torso. Isabella tugged, but the baby's head wouldn't come out. It was stuck above the cervix.

Isabella took me aside. She quietly explained to me that the baby had had hydrocephalus; the skull was abnormally large due to fluid on the brain. There was only one way to save the woman: we would have to separate the baby's body from its head. Once we had done that, I would have to reach inside the mother and crush the skull so that it could pass through the cervix.

I didn't want to let Isabella down, but I was horrified. 'I can't do that,' I told her. 'I can't.'

'You have to,' she replied calmly. Her hands were too small to grasp the skull. I looked down at my own large hands. I really didn't think I had it in me.

I watched as she performed the surgical procedure to remove the baby's head from its body. The baby didn't look human, but I was still shaken by it. In that moment, any vague idea I had had about studying midwifery was gone. It would have been a useful skill to complement my paediatric experience, but I clearly didn't have the stomach for it.

I stepped forward when Isabella instructed me and reached inside the woman's uterus. The patient was barely conscious now. I could feel the skull inside her womb, but I couldn't get hold of it. The more I tried, the more it slipped out of my grasp. *Fuck.* Isabella worked around me, trying to stem the bleeding, but time was running out. The skull was just too big; we couldn't remove it.

Isabella decided to try to perform surgery, though we had almost no equipment, no anaesthetic, no surgical table. We would have to transfer the patient to a small Catholic mission that was an hour down the road—the nuns had a surgical table.

We managed to get the mother in the LandCruiser, but we didn't make it to our destination. Mercifully, sadly, she died while we were in transit.

People often talk about the value of life in Africa, the idea that life is somehow worth less over there. Life is life, it's precious no matter where you live, but the people I worked with in South Sudan were more pragmatic about death than the people I grew up with. They didn't have the luxury of feeling any other way.

After Isabella left South Sudan, before her replacement was recruited, I was called into the maternity ward to help with another difficult birth. The baby was born, a little girl, but she was severely deformed. She had a cleft palate, she was blind and her vagina was malformed. A child would have struggled in Western society with that level of disability, let alone in South Sudan.

After the birth, we considered our options. We could fly the infant to Loki, where they could maybe start the process of surgery to mend the cleft palate. It would take more than one procedure. The baby's urethra didn't seem to have an opening, and there didn't seem to be any urine output, but maybe that could be fixed, too. We would need to keep her alive for a few days to monitor her, but she was hypothermic and we didn't have a humidicrib, so we used aluminium foil and cotton wool, warmed in the sun, as a crude emergency blanket. We waited to see if the baby had any urine or faecal output.

I arrived home from a water and sanitation session in the field to find the nursing team obviously upset. The mother had decided to take the baby home and the nurses couldn't convince her otherwise. She was totally impassive when I spoke to her; she had already formulated a plan. 'I will take the baby home and put it in the river,' she told me.

I asked the senior midwife to translate for me because I needed to understand exactly what the woman was thinking. The midwife explained that the mother was going to put the baby in the river, like Moses in the Bible. She said if God wanted the child to live, it would live. If not, God would call the baby home.

In South Sudan, a girl was an investment. Girls were raised to be married off for a bridal price. Boys cost money, but they would care for their parents in old age. Families were carefully calibrated, not for wealth and pleasure, but for survival. The mother looked at me very clearly and spoke. The midwife translated. 'This baby can't see. It can't eat. It can't have sex. It will not have babies. What good is it? We cannot afford it.'

I didn't know what to say. The mother was calm and completely detached. She hadn't bonded with the baby, deliberately. She was thinking of her other two children at home; she had her whole family to consider. A severely disabled child would drain their resources and put them all under threat. Who was I to tell her what to do? There was no guarantee that the baby would not die of dehydration or starvation in the coming days, anyway.

The local midwives were very distressed. They wanted the white woman to come in and take command, to tell the mother she had to save the child at any cost, but it wasn't my place. I couldn't imagine the challenges that this mother had faced every day just to stay alive. I asked her to care for the baby as well as she could, knowing full well that she intended to let her die, and then I told her she was free to leave.

This decision made the most sense to me at the time. I'm still not sure if it was the right thing to do.

# 5

# THAT ESCALATED QUICKLY

On a Friday night in Yirol, I would send one of our local staff members to the market to buy a goat. It cost seven Australian dollars to buy a live goat and whoever had gone to buy it would then butcher it for us at the compound. We kept the ribs and the legs. The staff member got to keep the head, the feet, the innards and also the skin, which they dried out and used to create baskets for babies. Mothers would hang the baskets from the branch of an acacia tree while they worked in the field.

Every Friday, I would fill half of a forty-gallon drum with hot coals, then marinate the goat meat and throw it onto the fire. I'd sit beside the pit eating Pringles and sipping Coke while I waited for it to cook. I thought it was quite a positive social thing, having a weekly barbecue, but the rest of the team weren't that enthusiastic about it. They struggled to understand why I would want to sit next to a makeshift barbecue in 35-degree heat in South Sudan, so they stayed in the comfort of their rooms while I did the ritual roasting. They were very happy to eat the goat; they just didn't want to sweat over it.

After a few Fridays passed, our head logistician, a local man named Julian, came to me wracked with guilt. He was very sheepish, could barely look me in the eyes. 'We can't keep buying the goat for you, Amanda. I am sorry.'

'That's okay, but why?'

'The boys are cheating you. I must put a stop to it. You give them money to buy the best goat, but they give you only the bones.'

'Oh, I see.' It would have been very rude to laugh. I had to explain instead that the feet and innards weren't really what we preferred to eat and since I wasn't keen to kill the goat myself, I thought it was a fair deal. This was quite the revelation for Julian but it prompted a suggestion. If I didn't want the 'best bits' we should share them more equally with the staff. Hence the first 'employee of the week' meat raffle was launched in Yirol.

One Friday evening, a staff member led a new goat into the compound, fresh from the market, but I could see out of the corner of my eye that its belly was sagging. The animal was clearly pregnant.

'Woah, what are you doing?' I shouted.

'This was the only goat in the market,' he told me.

It was hunger season and people were desperate, so they were selling whatever they had, including their precious pregnant animals. I like to eat meat, but this was a bit much. We couldn't take an animal from a desperate farmer and we weren't going to kill a pregnant goat, at least not on my watch. We ended up keeping the goat until it gave birth and then gave the kid to one of our local staff members, a special 'grand prize' for our employee of the month.

Victor learned the hard way how valuable animals are in South Sudan—some more valuable than others. He had flown out to a remote site to run a clinic for a day and he had managed to get himself into some trouble, so he radioed in for some intel.

'Amanda, I need to know the price of a donkey,' he said.

'You what?'

'How much does a donkey cost? It's an emergency.'

I leaned my head out of the office window and consulted with our local staff.

'A donkey? Fifty thousand Sudanese pounds,' they told me.

I relayed the info to Victor and he signed off, not bothering to explain himself. Shortly afterward, he called in again. 'Sorry, I need the price of a trick donkey.'

'What the hell is a trick donkey?'

'Just ask, will you?'

I stuck my head out of the window again and consulted the team.

'Ah, a trick donkey! A trick donkey is seventy thousand pounds.'

Victor thanked me again, and was silent for the better part of an hour. He checked in again just as they were taking off.

'So what's going on?' I asked.

'Well, we hit a donkey on the airstrip. It was messy . . . and the community was very upset because it was a special donkey.'

Victor explained that a trick donkey was trained to pull a plough.

'Right,' I laughed. 'So how's the plane? Is the propeller okay?'

'Uh, yeah, kind of,' Victor hesitated. 'It's full of donkey meat.'

Complacency was a problem in the field. After six months living in South Sudan, I felt like I had a good handle on the place, but I was still an outsider. And if I didn't fully understand that, then a useful lesson was headed my way.

Leo the hydrologist left our team just over halfway through my mission. A Kenyan engineer was trained to replace him but he was moved to a water project in Darfur, leaving me on my own to manage the entire water and sanitation program in Yirol. This meant wrapping my head around the mechanics of drilling a well. The local drill team did most of the work, I just needed a basic understanding, and for that there were more books in the Red Cross office.

As the program manager, in the eyes of the community I was responsible for the local drill team. It didn't strike me as a particularly onerous responsibility—I had been having a great time with the hygiene promotion team—but it seems I under-estimated what it meant. One day, I was paid a visit by one of the local soldiers, a major with an opposition group. The group was stationed in Yirol, where they would hold power until the country formalised its independence, and the major was a familiar face around the village, always recognisable because of his brightly coloured footwear.

The major came to our office one day and told me that a guy in the local drilling team had slept with his wife. According to local law, this person owed the major seven cows, but the adulterer had not paid, so the major had come to take our radio equipment in lieu of the cows because the adulterer was associated with the Red Cross. The radio equipment was our only connection to the Red Cross base in Lokichogio, so I had to do some fast talking to keep it in the building. I assured the major that I would speak to the person, that everything would be set right.

'I'll take care of it,' I told him.

I would soon find out that this was the wrong thing to say.

I spoke to the local driller who had reportedly slept with the major's wife and he assured me that the cow debt was already paid.

A couple of days later, I was out on the airstrip helping the medical team to run a tetanus vaccination program. I was working with Isabella's replacement, an older woman named Marta, who came from a small mountain village in Switzerland. She was much more adapted to ice climbing than the soaring African summer. She struggled with the heat. Marta was an excellent midwife, but an especially hot day would make her melt and she'd nap in the LandCruiser with the air-conditioning on. We started to implement siestas so she could make it through the day.

On this particular day, the team had vaccinated over eight hundred women. Marta and I packed the vaccination gear into the truck when we were done and drove down the street away from the airfield, towards the Red Cross compound. As we drove, we heard gunshots coming from the market. This was very unusual. We rounded a corner into the main street, preparing to reverse into the compound per normal security protocols (the cars always had to be facing outwards) and came face-to-face with a minor stampede—people running away from the market.

I instinctively pushed Marta's head towards the car seat. Behind us, the security team was ready, the compound gates wide open, their arms waving hysterically to usher us inside. I glanced back at them, then forward towards the market, where the source of all the trouble came into view. Less than 150 metres away, the major was marching down the street in his coloured footwear, shooting his AK-47 into the air.

I threw the truck in reverse, steering us backwards into the compound and hollering at the security guards to close the gate. The radio communications had lit up, in the meantime. The rest of the expat team was already inside the compound, sheltering in the kitchen pantry, now officially our safe room, and Marta and I ran through the compound to join them.

The pantry was a cement room with a wooden door, with locks on the inside—only one way in. The team had already called Loki on the satellite phone to let them know things had kicked off. The local staff were outside of the compound, in contact via radio. While we waited, listening to gunfire, they kept us up to date with the action. The major was looking for me, they said.

'Me?' I was confused. 'Why me?'

It turned out that when I had told the major that I would take care of it, he had interpreted this as *I will take on the debt.*

We sat in the pantry for a very long time, getting updates from the local staff. The expat team discussed the situation and we agreed that we should grab our runaway bags—emergency packs that included our passports, money and some essential items. They were on the back of the door in everyone's room. I didn't think there was much danger in going to grab them, so I volunteered, hustled out of the pantry, and raced from one bedroom to another, scooping up the bags. I always wondered how effective the standard issue runaway bag would be. They came with half a dozen condoms, not for what was known in the sector as 'emergency sex', but to carry water. I had tried it one day, carrying water in a condom. They can hold up to six litres before they burst.

While I made my rounds, I kept a close ear on the radio chatter from the local staff. When I got back to the safe room, I found Victor with a bread knife trying to carve a hole in the flyscreen that covered the safe room window. In my absence, they had decided that they would need an escape route if things escalated. Emotions were running a little high.

Eventually, the gunfire settled completely, but we were instructed by Loki to stay put overnight, so I went back to the bedrooms to grab some pillows and mattresses. We ate a pizza by candlelight, waiting for more news. We wouldn't have had a clue what was happening if the local team hadn't kept us up to date by radio.

By morning, we were being evacuated. A plane was coming from Lokichogio and we were tasked with getting our stuff together. This was bad news for the hospital and for the community, as services would disappear overnight. It was bad news for the local staff, too. If the Red Cross pulled out of Yirol, their jobs evaporated. The town officials begged us not to leave; they assured us it was safe, but we had no choice. Head office said go, so we went. Seemed a little over the top to me. It was all clearly a bit of a misunderstanding.

Back in Loki, during the security debrief, my team turned on each other. I thought everyone had been quite calm in the pantry—it was almost like a slumber party—but it turned out that they were really frightened, and irritated with me. When I had left the storage room with the radio, they had had no idea what was happening.

I was puzzled by their response to the situation. I was the one running around the compound grabbing their bags and mattresses. I hadn't felt particularly alarmed by it, so I didn't see why they should. I knew that people responded to stress differently, but we were working in a conflict zone. Wasn't this all part of the deal?

The head of Red Cross field operations wanted to fly back into Yirol a couple of days later to see if the organisation could re-establish itself in the area. He asked if I would go along with him and I was more than keen. I wanted to apologise to the major for the confusion about the cows. I was also worried about the staff we had left behind.

We got a hero's welcome when the plane touched down. The local army general assured us that everything was fine now and we were welcome back. The local driller had paid the adultery debt and the major was safely imprisoned.

'Do you want to see him?' the general asked.

The major was sitting outside the barracks, still wearing his coloured footwear. A pair of handcuffs attached his ankle to the leg of the bamboo chair he was sitting on. If he'd stood up and lifted the chair an inch off the ground, the cuff would have slipped off the chair leg and he could have walked free. But anyway, he seemed happy to sit.

'Hello, Amanda!' he called when he saw me.

'Hey, major, how are you?'

'I'm so sorry about the other day,' he replied. 'I didn't mean to frighten you.'

We had a good chat and the major assured us that it was all a big misunderstanding. The Red Cross was safe in Yirol and he hoped we would all come back soon. We thanked him, it was good to hear. The field security manager was satisfied.

'I do have something very important to discuss with you before you go,' the major said.

'What's that?' the security manager replied.

'Technically I am now a prisoner of war,' the major explained. 'Will the Red Cross be coming to visit me? Because I'd really like a tennis ball and some cigarettes.'

Technically he wasn't actually a prisoner of war, but we brought him cigarettes anyway.

It was extraordinary how fast the market grew while I was in Yirol. When I first arrived, there was virtually nothing. Vendors would sell Maggi stock cubes by the individual cube. Salt and sugar would be sold in individual serves, and there were sometimes second-hand clothes for sale. But as the peace process was nutted out between the opposition group and the Sudanese government, the borders opened and people started moving goods into South Sudan. This had a bizarre effect on the Sudanese fashion scene, if nothing else.

In preparation for the signing of the peace agreement in January 2005, the Sudan People's Liberation Movement (SPLM) passed a law that no one could be naked in the market. When independence was formalised, South Sudan would be a civilised nation, which meant that people must wear clothes. An entrepreneurial man set up a second-hand clothing rental store on the outskirts of Yirol so that visitors coming into the market could avoid breaking the law. Villagers would stop off, grab an assortment of stylish 1960s fashion and then drop the items back to the vendor when their business was done in town. As it happened, most of the items available for rent were dresses, but that didn't stop the Dinka men from wearing them. Pants, dresses and gendered colours had no meaning for the South Sudanese, which was very charming. Young Dinka warriors, tall and lean with twelve-pack abs, would stroll into town in polyester house dresses and velvet hats, looking very pleased with themselves. At one point, nail polish found its way into the market and the men started getting around with pink and electric blue nails.

Clothing was a symbol of power and wealth in one of the poorest nations in the world. Towards the end of my mission, I was negotiating for a new water point with a tribal chief who desperately wanted to form a new city. The peace agreement had been signed, discussions were underway for the establishment of South Sudan as an independent country, and the chief was inspired to contribute to the new enthusiasm for 'nation building'. You couldn't have a city if you didn't have water, he argued, so the four water points that we had agreed to install in the surrounding area (where all the people lived) should be moved to the crossroads under the chief's dominion. They would build a market and a 'shopping centre' and the people would follow—kind of a *Field of Dreams* theory of urban planning. The chief would be in charge of South Sudan's newest city, but several hundred people in surrounding villages would go without a water supply in the meantime.

I met with the chief several times and each time he was naked except for a string of beads around his waist, and a polyester sheet draped over one shoulder. Each time we met, he came with a retinue of bodyguards, very fierce and handsome young men who also happened to be naked, except for the guns they carried. We would all sit together, cross-legged under the trees and discuss his vision for the city. They were all naked and I wasn't, but I rarely noticed how they were (or weren't) dressed. Nudity was common in South Sudan and my eyes never wandered. At least, not until the chief got his hands on some clothes.

After several meetings, the decision had been made in Yirol: we would drill water points as planned, where the population was now, not where they may move to in the future. I had to go and tell the chief that his hope for a mega-city might be delayed, and I arrived to find the elderly man wearing a pair of red silk panties. He had been to the new market in Yirol and had found a supply of women's underwear, and his bodyguards were decked out in the same apparel, though their colours were aqua and black.

Greetings were more enthusiastic than usual and the chief had me take photos of his newly outfitted crew. They posed proudly next to their best cows, lined up in women's underwear like they were wearing new tuxedos. It was kind of fantastic, until we sat down.

I was on my way to a water consultation meeting one day when I was flagged down by the driver of a semi-trailer. He told me he had a wounded man on his truck, perched up on top of the cargo. When I climbed up there, I found a man with a blanket around his waist and a huge pool of blood between his legs. My first thought was that someone had cut off his genitalia, but then he raised his hand and I saw the real wound, a huge hole in the middle of his palm. It was amazing. I could see right through to the other side. Bizarrely, the guy could still move his fingers.

The truck driver and his men managed to carry the wounded man down to the side of the road, where I did my best to treat him. I was struggling to dress the wound and tape an IV drip to his slick, sweating skin when my patient announced that he had to go to the toilet.

'Jesus, can he wait?' I asked my team. He assured them that he couldn't.

In the end, I had to station myself next to the patient, holding his wounded arm and the IV drip in the air, and looking off at the horizon while he used his good hand to hold his penis and urinate. If I had been paying closer attention, I might have seen that the patient was going to pass out. Instead, I felt a jolt of dead weight as he slipped out of my grasp and crashed to the ground, peeing in a golden arc as he fell. Most of the urine hit my leg.

Oddly, that wasn't my fondest memory involving wee in South Sudan. There was another moment that I will never forget, which started out quite grimly. While out working with one of the communities, I noticed a little boy squatting to urinate and milking his penis, clearly having some trouble. I asked his mother about his symptoms, but the odd urination ritual was the only real problem. He struggled to pee. It was painful for the little boy, and on top of that, the other kids in the village were making fun of him.

On my next weekend away in Loki, I asked the head surgeon from the Red Cross hospital to fly the kid out for an examination. Tests revealed that the little boy had a golf ball-sized build-up of calcium in his bladder, a side-effect of sickle cell anaemia. The surgeon couldn't do much about the sickle cell, but he removed the calcium deposit and corrected the urine retention. The boy had a terminal prognosis in the long term, but in the meantime, he recovered well from the surgery.

I met the boy and his grandfather when the plane landed in Yirol, and drove them back to the village myself. When I returned with the little patient, the whole village turned up to meet him. The boy didn't run to his parents, he positioned himself next to the Red Cross truck as the village gathered around. There was huge excitement building. When the crowd had assembled, the boy put his hand up to quieten everyone. He took a good long look at his audience, then pulled his pants down and planted his hands on his hips. With a huge grin on his face, he pissed right where he was standing—a beautiful, clear, strong stream of wee. And the crowd went nuts.

Late one morning, we got word of a tribal conflict that had left many injured men out of reach, in a remote area to the north of Yirol. The SPLM requested that we go out to attend to the wounded, but we were severely understaffed. The majority of the expat team had flown to Lokichogio for their rostered weekend break, leaving me and a Kenyan midwife named Rose behind with a German nurse who was in Yirol for a supervision visit. I radioed in to the Red Cross base in Loki for advice and they gave us permission to go and retrieve the wounded, but not until the following day. It would be two full days since the conflict by the time we got there. I was worried about what we'd find when we arrived.

We set out in two Red Cross LandCruisers early on a Sunday morning, with the proviso that we would turn around no later than 3 p.m. Tight security protocols were in place for the trip and Lokichogio would be monitoring our progress hourly. We had to be back in Yirol before dark.

There were no road maps or GPS leading us to the conflict. We drove out with only the vaguest idea of where the skirmish had taken place, and eventually spied two plumes of black smoke on the horizon. We drove towards them, coming to stop in a nearby village. There we were told that the two warring parties had separated and made camp in the bush with their wounded, so the German nurse and I decided to separate as well. We'd each drive out towards a different camp, then reconvene in the village.

I set off with one of the best drivers we had. We were driving across the bumpy terrain of a dry lakebed, through grass and heavy smoke, where the path seemed like nothing but a series of deep potholes. We bounced through them as though we were on a trampoline. My driver told me they were elephant tracks, but I hadn't seen a single elephant in South Sudan in the many months that I had been here. The local staff had told me that they were all eaten during the war. As we reached the other side of the plain, the smoke cleared and I saw what we were really driving through. Dead bodies began appearing by the side of the road.

It was carnage. The bodies were sparse at first, but as we reached the spot where the main battle had taken place, they increased. The skirmish had happened two days earlier, but I wondered if I should stop and check that these people were actually dead. Just ahead, I thought I saw a man moving in the grass, and I asked my driver to stop the car, grabbing my first-aid kit. As I got closer, I realised that it was another corpse, severely bloated, the stomach heavily distended.

I wanted to bury the bodies, or at least cover them, but it was getting close to three o'clock. There were wounded people still waiting, so we left the dead where they lay.

When we arrived at the camp, I found almost twenty men in need of treatment, many of them with small calibre gunshot wounds. They were such tiny holes; it was hard to imagine the internal damage. I couldn't possibly take them all. I leaped into action, swabbing everything I could with Betadine and trying to triage the patients, looking for the seven worst-off to take back to the clinic. We used coloured bands in the field for triage—it was too hard to remember faces when you were triaging mass trauma, so we gave the most urgent patients a red armband—but I didn't have them with me. When I found someone who needed to come back to the clinic, I gave him a handful of cotton wool to hold instead. I moved fast, mindful of the time, and the rubber gloves I wore quickly filled with sweat, which streamed down my arms while I worked.

I found a guy with a dislocated hip so I put him in the truck, and another man who had been shot in the face. The gunshot victim seemed fine—he was conscious and talking—but I couldn't wrap my head around the fact that a bullet had passed through his head. There was another man who had a compound leg fracture where a bullet had hit him—his shin bone was shattered and was protruding through the skin—so I did my best to splint his leg and loaded him into the car. I had IV fluids with me, but no time and no way to hang them. The best I could do was mix up a bottle of rehydration salts and pass it to the wounded men, signalling for them to drink.

I was clear-headed and methodical, but I knew time was getting away from me. The German nurse had radioed through to tell me she was back at the village. She hadn't made it to the second camp because there was no access road. It was late and she was nervous. I had to work faster.

When we set off, the car was completely full and everyone was sweating bullets. My pants were saturated, and my shirt clung to me. In the back, the wounded men were deathly quiet.

I had overloaded the LandCruiser. The men were clustered on bench seats, the man with the compound fracture stretched in between them, weighing down the chassis. All of a sudden, we hit a divot and the car was bogged. We couldn't move—each wheel seemed to be stuck in a perfectly sized hole. The only way I could inch us free was to jump up and down on the rear bumper, bouncing the wounded men viciously.

When we took off again, the second car came through on the radio. 'When you get to the village, don't stop,' she said. 'Soldiers are here and the atmosphere is tense.'

We agree to go through town at speed, falling in to convoy with the German nurse without stopping, taking a different road back to Yirol. It would be safer that way.

In the back of our vehicle, the guy with the fractured leg had lost his splint and his calf was at a right angle to the rest of his leg. He was too quiet. I was worried he was in shock and we were still an hour and a half away from Yirol. 'We have to stop,' I told our driver, but he said no, we were not safe. I trusted him, though I couldn't really understand why he was so stressed. I thought the fighting was over—we were simply providing aid. I didn't know we were driving through land that belonged to the losing side, or that the men in the car were their enemies.

At one point, we came upon a thick log that had been dragged across the road. The road ran through a dirt field, so there was nothing stopping us from driving around the obstruction, but to my driver this was a very bad sign. Someone was trying to block our path. He remained tense, minute after minute, until we were clear of the tribal lands.

The minute I saw him relax, I made him stop. I had to fix the leg splint and make sure the patients were drinking the rehydration salts. The German nurse stopped just ahead of us and jumped out to help with the wounded. We worked quickly, stabilising the leg and checking the patients, but it wasn't fast enough. Just as we were debating whether we should move some of the men into the other vehicle, we were surrounded.

The people came out of nowhere, a few of them carrying guns. I moved just fast enough to get inside the car and lock the doors, while the German nurse had raced to her own car. The villagers ignored her vehicle, which carried no patients, so I radioed her to drive away and wait at a safe distance.

The people surrounding us closed in, testing the doors and the windows. Most of them were unarmed, but they were very agitated, and the men in the back of the car were beginning to respond.

I got out of the car. I marched around to the driver's side, towards one of the armed men, and he came towards me. I started yelling at him, in English, and he yelled back, in Dinka. I was full of righteous fury, spouting the principles of my organisation. Not respecting wounded combatants was against the rules. How dare he disrespect the internationally recognised symbol of the Red Cross, et cetera. Obviously he didn't understand a word I was saying, and I had no idea what he was saying either.

All of a sudden, I felt a tap on my shoulder and I turned to face a huge man, about fifteen centimetres taller than me. He was carrying a gun. In perfectly clear English he said, 'You need to leave now. Get in the car and go. I will take care of this.'

I thought twice, looked at his gun, and pulled my shit together.

'Thank you,' I told him politely, walking quickly to the car door.

My driver was in shock and couldn't get the car moving, so I reached over and pressed his leg into the accelerator, slamming the horn to clear a path through the crowd. We started to move, catching up to the other Red Cross vehicle.

As South Sudan moved towards independence, the country changed rapidly, and it happened right before our eyes. Television arrived in Yirol towards the end of my mission, beamed in via satellite from every corner of the globe, and with it came this new global perspective, a sense of place in the world.

Just before I left, I was called to the army barracks to visit the general, who had recently seen some news coverage from Australia.

'We heard you worked with the Aboriginal people in Australia,' the general began.

'I did, yes.'

'You must tell us more about them,' he said.

'Right,' I answered. 'What would you like to know?'

'We watched a documentary on television last night about the Australian Aboriginals and it seems they are in a very bad way. We would like to know more about this.' The general explained that as South Sudan was going to be a new country, it was important for them to understand on which rung of the ladder they sat. 'It seems to us that we are not the poorest people in the world. Perhaps the Aboriginals are worse off than us?'

*That's a ridiculous proposition,* I wanted to tell him, but I could see how you'd get that impression.

# 6

## THERE IS NOTHING FUNNY ABOUT TSUNAMI

When I got back from South Sudan, I went for debriefing in Melbourne. Charlotte, the field personnel manager, was there to meet me, to see how I had got on. I went through the normal debrief procedures, which included being asked if I would be interested in another mission. My response was automatic: 'Of course! It was fantastic.'

'Great,' she replied. 'We'll call you in about three months.'

'Three months?! You're kidding me.' I was ready to head straight back out there.

Charlotte gave me a very measured look and reminded me that it was standard practice in the Red Cross to have at least three months off between missions. It was important to do normal things; to connect with friends and family. I also needed to give my body a break after a year of hard living conditions.

I was sent to a psychologist for a mental health debrief, which was meant to help me process being back in my normal world. It was familiar but also like an alien planet. Why was the supermarket so big? Why was there so much choice? Was there really a need for thirty-two different types of cereal? I just wanted one, and I didn't really care what it was.

I struggled to connect with people, although I tried not to let it show. People would ask me how everything went on my mission, but it was mostly out of politeness. Within five minutes the conversation would swing off to nappies, the cost of petrol, the weather and whatever else people worry about in their day-to-day lives. I didn't have a problem with this, in principle, because I didn't feel the need to talk about my work in any detail, but it was hard to contribute to the conversation. I was completely out of touch.

The psychologist gave me a great piece of advice. She told me to ask a friend to put copies of *Woman's Day* and *Who* magazine aside for me while I was away on a mission. When I got back, I could flick through them and pick up a few conversation starters. This worked a treat when Britney Spears shaved her head.

'What about bald Britney Spears? How crazy was that?!'

In later years, the friend who was tasked with keeping me in the loop started cutting and pasting major celebrity news stories into emails. And eventually, the internet caught up with the humanitarian world. If I want to read about Britney Spears now, I can do it in real time.

Meanwhile, the three-month break after South Sudan felt like it lasted three seconds, and I was much better off for it. When I meet people starting out in this line of work, I recommend they take at least three months off between missions. It's advice I wish I had followed more in my own career.

During my downtime, I did a couple of short stints of remote area nursing and took a short course for my master's degree, including a subject on disaster management. Everyone in the course kept talking about Aceh. *Aceh* this and *Aceh* that. I felt like an idiot—what the fuck was Aceh? Eventually, I just asked. They looked at me like I was from the moon.

'Banda Aceh.'

'. . .?'

'The tsunami?'

Banda Aceh, on the coast of Indonesia, was the closest major city to the epicentre of the 2004 Boxing Day earthquake, and was absolutely devastated by the tsunami that followed. Over 160,000 people were killed in the region and the city was reduced to a pile of rubble. Toxic waste was dumped over the land, tens of thousands of people were displaced and bodies decomposing in the streets were buried in mass graves, all of which had made news headlines across the globe. Banda Aceh was synonymous with the tsunami, but this fact had somehow passed me by. We had been so out of touch in South Sudan, and the news came in so late and in such a piecemeal way, that no single place had managed to make an impression.

It was sort of ironic, then, that my next posting for the Red Cross was to Banda Aceh. I got called up for the mission on the second-to-last day of my course, a very high-profile posting under the circumstances. I enjoyed telling my class that I would be there in seven days.

I was heading to a small island called Simeulue off the west coast of Indonesia to do some first-aid training. The island had been hit so hard by the tsunami that it had literally tilted, leaving reefs exposed as they stuck out of the water. I was part of the rearguard of the humanitarian response, which is about training and prevention. The rescue effort had happened in the first seventy-eight hours; by ten months post-tsunami, when I arrived, the rebuilding work was well under way. My project was to support the community to be better prepared for the next disaster, to teach them how to help themselves before more help arrived. I was going to adapt the hygiene education program I had run in South Sudan to teach the Simeulue basic first aid, but first I was going to spend six weeks in Banda Aceh helping out with an infectious disease program.

The International Committee of the Red Cross had done a major assessment of all the camps for people displaced by the tsunami in Aceh and there was a serious concern that with the coming wet season there would be a disease outbreak of some kind. Malaria was always a huge threat, but they were particularly worried about cholera, and conditions were so poor in the camps that it was just a matter of time. A list of camps had been drawn up and various aid agencies had taken responsibility for them, including six camps that became the responsibility of the Australian Red Cross. I was embedded in that part of the organisation to try to stave off the coming outbreak. Again, I was meant to do hygiene promotion work, which meant teaching people to wash their hands. Basic hygiene and clean drinking water was our best defence against disease.

From the air, you could see the incredible destruction the wave had caused. There was a crashed plane by the side of the Banda Aceh airport, which had come down during the first response effort, blocking the runway; driving into town all I saw was rubble. Occasionally, a lone wall would be standing amid the piles of broken bricks and twisted metal, or some random neighbour-hood pocket would appear relatively unscathed, but there was no way you could tell what Banda Aceh had looked like before the wave hit. Even after months of rebuilding, most of the city looked post-apocalyptic.

The day after I arrived, I had a meeting at the ministry of health in the centre of town. I noticed a line painted on the wall in the foyer, maybe two metres above the ground, and I asked my escort what it was. 'Watermark,' he said. *Unbelievable.* We were twenty minutes' drive away from the coast and the building had been submerged in two metres of water when the wave hit. At least it was still standing.

Banda Aceh is an Islamic region, and most of the mosques were still standing, too. The local people said it was Allah's work. Maybe they were right, but people don't skimp on cement or quality materials when they're building a house of worship. That might have had something to do with it, too.

Around the coast, you saw nothing but the cement foundations of the houses that once stood there. The houses had been obliterated, just washed away. Usually, all that was left was the squat toilet and the *mandi*, the cement water reserve that sat beside the toilet in countries where you pour rather than flush. In certain places, 200–300 metres of land had been reclaimed by the ocean. At low tide, you could see waves breaking around the remains of houses that had been lost to the sea.

The tsunami response operation was massive. It was estimated that over twenty-two thousand Red Cross staff and volunteers had been deployed to the affected regions in the first three months. Even now, ten months later, there were thousands of Red Cross personnel still on tsunami missions, with over twenty different National Societies providing support. In Aceh, it meant we used up a lot of office space and accommodation in a city that had essentially been destroyed.

The Red Cross movement took over virtually a whole street filled with opulent houses that had once belonged to oil industry representatives working in the area. Spread across seven or eight mansions, the various National Societies worked, collaborated and coordinated activities to respond to the needs of the community in Aceh. The Federation, which was there to coordinate activities, had a huge house right in the middle, a ridiculous palace filled with overstuffed couches and fake chandeliers, and a sweeping staircase that led up to a series of bedroom offices. It was opulence, Indonesian-style, where plastic stood in for glass and the tiles were all a sick peach colour, but it was a lot more impressive than what I was used to. There were no tiles at all in Yirol.

I expected a frenetic pace, but the response effort was transitioning to recovery and development, which meant building capacity in the local population. Some of the Aussies in my team were setting up a local ambulance service and another team was working on creating a blood bank, and most people were there on twelve-month contracts rather than fast, furious rotations. The pace was calm and steady, because there was less urgency, and the humanitarian community had settled into a fairly relaxed lifestyle. There was an alcohol ban because Aceh was ruled by Sharia law, but in the privacy of their homes people found their way around it.

The Red Cross was only part of the picture. There were nearly two hundred and fifty aid organisations in Aceh when I arrived and thousands of expats working in-country. We tried to work in a coordinated way, but everyone had their own mission and agenda. Even within the Red Cross, the work was quite fragmented, as everyone scrambled to allocate the millions in donations that had poured in when the disaster hit.

In the wider circle of aid organisations, things were even more haphazard. Only fifty or so of the organisations working in Aceh had plans that were approved by the local government and there was no formal cluster system to make sure all the humanitarian projects were efficient and complementary. We didn't know what anyone else was doing, although it was obvious that they were all doing something. We saw their branded vehicles and logos all over town.

The first displaced persons' camp that I went to assess was covered in stickers from other organisations. The bins had Care stickers on them, the portable toilets had Concern Worldwide stickers, the tents had UNICEF logos on them. There was branding on everything, but no one seemed to be taking care of anything. The water tanks were empty, despite the Oxfam stickers on them. Little kids were bathing in fetid water, right next to exposed sewage from overflowing toilets.

When I asked the people living in the camps where the other aid organisations were, they said they hadn't seen anyone in months. In the first wave of the tsunami response, everyone did whatever they could to build these temporary camps but then the organisations moved on to the next phase of aid work, building permanent housing. There was nothing sexy or urgent about the refugee camps anymore and they had been allowed to fall into ruin.

The first camp I looked at was based in a sawmill, which had been operational before the tsunami hit. There were 200 people living there; roughly fifty families had erected tents in and around the commercial logging equipment. These families were all that was left of a large coastal community south of Banda Aceh, and the average family size had shrunk from six or seven people down to one or two. The survivors had walked together from the coast into Banda Aceh, in search of a new life. Looking around, I saw a lot of single men and teenagers. The older people had been killed, the small children had been killed and many of the mothers were gone, too.

I was aware, as I travelled from camp to camp, that people were suffering from assessment fatigue. I was just the latest in a long line of well-meaning humanitarian workers who were asking questions and taking photographs. The questions were always the same: *What do you need? Who did you lose? How many people are in your family?* Unfortunately, many of those well-meaning people never came back; the information just got absorbed somewhere. I felt an uneasiness in the camps, a wariness. It was almost like I was a tourist, and they were sick of being a spectacle.

Things are different now—there are online platforms where all this information is shared—but back then I had to carry the clipboard, ask the questions and take the photographs in order to make an assessment and justify how I was going to move forward. What I tried to do, remembering the advice I got when I landed in Sudan, was to keep my mouth shut and my eyes open.

The people living in the sawmill didn't want to go back to their devastated land, but the sawmill operators wanted them out. It made sense because the building industry in Aceh was booming, but it was terrible news for the villagers. I actually thought it was for the best. From a disease control point of view, I wanted to get them out of there, too. Teaching people to wash their hands was unnecessary—the community members were observant Muslims who washed five times a day—but I couldn't stop them from getting sick when the environment around them was rotten. There were no toilets, there were too many drainage problems in the sawmill and all the tents were mouldy and getting holes. These people didn't need a hygiene promotion program, they needed to be relocated.

The other camps that the Australian Red Cross had taken on were not much better off. One of them was on the grounds of

Banda Aceh University, which had to be cleared out before school started back in two months. Another was built on a flood plain on top of an old rice paddy. In the months since the tsunami, some of the people had been moved from tents to temporary structures called long-houses. A few of the camps did have toilets built, but the faeces had risen to ground level and the wooden slats over the drop holes were broken. The plastic sheeting around the toilets was torn, which made them very unsafe for women, and people had started defecating openly at night-time, wherever they could find space.

The Federation of the Red Cross was developing a major housing project in Aceh at this time, a fund for 200,000 prefabricated houses that could be assembled like a Meccano set; ten people could put a house together in one day. Meanwhile, there was a mandate from the Indonesian government banning aid agencies from distributing any more tents, even though the existing tents were falling apart. The government wanted people in permanent housing as fast as possible.

The Federation houses were meant to be erected on the land that people already owned, where their original houses had once stood, but the sea had risen substantially along the coast and many of those original blocks were gone. There were no records, so new maps had to be drawn up, based on conversations with the local community. How did you prove who owned what? Where should the disappeared blocks be relocated? If you were renting and we built you a house on the old parcel of land, did it belong to you or your landlord? And was it an aid organisation's responsibility to rebuild three houses that a wealthy landowner had lost? All of this stuff had to be negotiated, dragging out the process, which left a little window of crisis that the Australian Red Cross had to manage. We estimated that it would take two years for the permanent housing to go in, but the people in my camps needed to be moved immediately.

I started talking to my bosses about a change of direction. We needed to help the communities in our care move and we had the funds to do it, so we turned our focus from hygiene education to a transition shelter project. I was twenty-nine years old and I had no experience in the area, so I was just going to steer things initially until a project manager came on board. We needed carpenters, builders, a whole squadron of labourers, and an engineer to guide them. The idea was to build temporary settlements that met a basic standard of hygiene, as quickly as we could. When the project manager arrived and put a team together, I would move on to Simeulue per the original plan and teach people how to apply bandages, like a normal nurse would.

'Do whatever you can in the meantime,' I was told. *Do whatever it takes.*

My experience in South Sudan was incredibly useful when it came to figuring out what the displaced communities would need. The planning phase of the project involved sitting down and asking questions, letting the local people lead the conversation. This is how we learned, for example, that the women felt much safer when the toilet doors opened inwards—they could hold them closed, even if the lock was broken. The few toilets that were clean in the various camps I'd visited had been allocated to specific families, which told us that ownership and control had an impact on the general level of hygiene.

What I couldn't learn from the communities, I had to research. With so many development and aid agencies in Aceh, I had a wealth of experts within arm's reach, and a library of education materials on hand. While a lot of the other expats were out partying, I studied. I read documents about building refugee camps and learned about the Sphere Standards, the globally accepted standards for humanitarian assistance. They dictated how many water points should be built in a camp per number of people, and how many toilets, with guidelines for camp structure and management. It was all laid out very clearly. All I had to do was stick to the guidelines, or tweak them where necessary to suit the communities and the sites that we had to manage.

I needed an engineer but I didn't have time to go through a long recruitment process, so I asked around until a name came up. A local woman by the name of Cut was recommended by the Canadian Red Cross engineer as a good potential candidate, which was good enough for me. Cut was very tiny, mild-mannered but determined; she turned my whole image of a Muslim woman on its head. She was a civil engineer, a working mother of two, and she drove her own car, though she also wore a headscarf and was very observant in her religion. She had a lot of experience and she was very keen to help.

Cut had been at home with her children when the tsunami hit. Her husband was outside when the wave struck and washed him away. She was washed out of the house by the force of the wave, but she had managed to cling to her two children, sheltering with them inside a water tank at the top of a 15-metre tower. They were stranded up there for hours until the water level came down and Cut was able to go in search of her husband. She found him in the Red Cross hospital, still alive, three days later. She had been wanting to work with the Red Cross ever since.

Everyone in Banda Aceh had a horrific story, if you asked. In a very detached and pragmatic way, a father would tell you about the child who had been washed out of his grasp. You would hear about bodies found on rooftops, or bodies never found at all. One man I worked with had left his wedding party to get some ice when the wave hit. Everyone at the wedding had been killed except for his fiancée, who was getting ready for the ceremony in another house.

People had lost so much, but that wasn't the first story they wanted to tell you. They talked about where they were now and where they wanted to be. The man who lost his family at the wedding now worked twelve hours a day trying to help other people who had been affected. Like everyone else I met, his primary focus was how to make things better.

Maybe it was just a matter of timing. I'm sure things would have looked very different in the immediate aftermath of the disaster, but when I arrived in Aceh, people were generally quite happy and welcoming. They didn't see themselves as victims, especially our local team. They were the lucky ones who had survived (with thanks to Allah, they usually said). They firmly believed it was their job to move forward and rebuild, and everybody was looking for an opportunity to do that. Obviously the community had been deeply traumatised, but on a day-to-day level it was cohesive and determined. People really wanted to bounce back.

I began building the first settlement within weeks of arriving in Banda Aceh, a transitional housing site for 150 families that were living in tents and long-houses along the Aceh Besar coast, about thirty minutes' drive from the city. These people wanted to stay close to their land so that when the officials came through to register people for permanent housing, they would be there to stake their claim. But the site presented a few problems for me: it was full of rubble and potholes, and much of it was still flooded. We'd have a hard time building anything that would last.

Cut came up with a workable idea: we'd build temporary housing on platforms. The no-tent rule was on the way in, but tents on raised wooden daises could work. We would use crushed coral to make pathways between the tents and build enough water points and toilets to keep everyone healthy. It would be glamping, essentially, or something slightly less romantic, but it would do the job.

Cut took over site planning, marking out where each of the new structures would be erected, while I became an expert in septic toilet design. (I was up to my elbows in poo again, but more conceptually this time.) I also struck up a relationship with a Kiwi logistics company to get a team of tradies on board, and engaged the community itself in the project, which would provide the labour force. Relatively quickly, I had assembled a working unit that was ready to roll out the camp.

The engineers working in other arms of the Red Cross laughed at me, because I did everything the hard way and the most expensive way. I stuck rigorously to the Sphere guidelines, whereas they took a more efficient approach. They were building shelters, but I was specifically trying to prevent a disease outbreak, so if anything bothered me from a public health perspective, I had to get it fixed, I couldn't let it alone. And because I was told it would be two years until permanent housing was ready, I planned for two years. I didn't want the Red Cross associated with anything like the camps I had seen when I'd arrived. If we were going to put our name on something, it was going to last.

Within a few weeks, the first camp was finished. I was pretty proud. It looked like a rustic little resort, so I was surprised to find that the families that had worked with us in the planning and building of the new facilities were still living in their shitty old tents. In a meeting with the community leaders, we explained the handover process. The new site was ready to go, they could move in whenever they wanted, but we came back a few days later and the new tents were still empty. We called a community meeting.

The feedback was positive, the families had no complaints, they thanked us for all the hard work, but something was clearly not right. When the meeting ended, Cut and I milled around outside for some time, watching. It started to rain. I watched a man go into a mouldy, leaking tent with his three small children.

'I don't get it!' I told Cut in disbelief.

We turned to leave but the man waved us over and spoke to Cut in the local language, then motioned for us to look inside. There were buckets on the floor to catch the water streaming in from the roof, and the mould smelled terrible, but at the end of the tent there was a huge TV. The three kids were gathered around it watching *SpongeBob SquarePants*.

The family had rigged an electrical cable from a power source up the road, dragging electricity in on a bunch of precarious wires. Between the dodgy leads and the rain, someone was going to get electrocuted, I thought. But I got the message, loud and clear. The families weren't going to move unless we gave them power. You couldn't blame them—their lives were hard enough as it was. Electricity wasn't included in the Sphere guidelines but it was clearly necessary here.

We spent two or three weeks putting a lightbulb and a power point in each of the new tents and *boom*, mass migration, the families were in.

I arrived in Aceh in October 2005 and finished that first camp in November, then in December I was told that the media were coming for the one-year anniversary of the disaster. AusAID, the foreign aid arm of the Australian government, was sending twenty journalists from home to witness the recovery efforts. People wanted to see where their donations were going; they wanted to feel good about their contribution.

Everyone was nervous. The response effort wasn't going as fast as anyone would have liked, but the complications of working in the biggest disaster in half a century posed unforeseeable problems and delays. Everyone was working their arses off, but if there was a backlash in public opinion because people decided the money wasn't being spent fast enough, it could seriously hurt the Red Cross's reputation.

As I came to learn over the following years, when in doubt, hold a meeting. The senior management called us together and told us that we needed to show progress. The blood bank project and the ambulance program were mostly conceptual at that point, the immediate relief work was well and truly over, and we were in a transition phase. There wasn't much to *show*. I was the newest member to the team and the youngest. Naively, I said, 'Can't we just explain why it takes so much time?' Everyone in the meeting groaned. Then they decided that my project would be the best example of work done in incredibly challenging circumstances.

'The journos will be tough on you,' the media manager warned me. 'People think we're not spending the money fast enough.' In order to prepare me for an onslaught of questions, he sent me thirty-two pages of key messages, which I read and forgot pretty much instantly.

In the lead-up to Boxing Day, the media flew in and I walked them around the camp. All the major Australian outlets turned up: broadsheet newspaper journalists, quite a few television crews, even a glossy magazine journalist. I explained all the issues that came with building back, showed them the changed coastline and the rubble and the house foundations inside the surf, and then introduced them to some of the beneficiaries that were living in the new settlement. It was all very pleasant and straightforward, I thought, no tricky questions. The landscape spoke more than any key messages. The journalists jotted down some notes and took off, and I went back to work thinking my job was done. But later the same afternoon, I got a call from head office. The glossy magazine that had a journalist wanted to write a feature story about me.

I won't tell you exactly how I felt about that; suffice to say I resisted. But the media manager at Australian Red Cross was adamant; we owed the magazine a favour. The magazine wanted to do 'a day in the life of Amanda McClelland'. I told them I'd give them an hour.

Over the preceding weeks, I had picked up an assistant, a little girl from the camp who had excellent English and helped me to translate when Cut wasn't around. Her parents had been killed, she was living with her uncle, and she'd started following me around whenever I was working. She was pretty cute. She was with me when the journalist came back, because I'd promised to take her to the dentist. It wasn't a very big deal—the kid had a cracked molar, which was going to cost me about twenty dollars to get fixed. An abscess would have formed if the tooth wasn't taken care of and the girl would have gotten quite sick, which would have been a bigger problem for me further down the line. I made an easy, practical choice.

The journalist loved this story, of course, and made it into the feature. The journalist was determined to portray me as a hero, so he took whatever he could get. He even had a photographer ready to capture the perfect hero shot and we spent about three hours trying to get it.

'We need a shot of you with the children!' the photographer announced. 'What about these guys?'

He grabbed a bunch of kids that I had literally never seen before and arranged them around me in the frame. I was so over it that I didn't argue—the sooner he got the pictures he wanted, the better.

'Right, I've gotta get back to work,' I announced, scattering kids as I stood up.

'No, wait. I need a shot of you on the beach! Give us half an hour more.'

We spent at least twenty minutes trying to find the most perfectly devastated beach on the coast of Aceh. When we got there, the photographer arranged me on some driftwood and told me to stare at the landscape and try to look serious. He had spent the six weeks prior to this sitting around the royal court in Copenhagen, waiting for Princess Mary to have a baby, and now he was trying to arrange my face at the right angle to catch a mournful glint of fading sunlight. It was ridiculous. 'Can you look out across the devastation?' he asked. I couldn't help myself, I started laughing.

The photographer looked at me sternly and said, 'Amanda, there is nothing funny about tsunami.'

I disagreed. I'd had a lot of fun working with the community. They loved to laugh. And besides that, the photographer was pretty fucking hilarious.

We negotiated with the local government to secure a parcel of land for the community that was living in the old sawmill. The site wasn't ideal, but it was better than nothing: 15 metres wide and 1.5 kilometres long, running along a bank of the Aceh River. Unfortunately, the location was already inhabited. While digging a hole for one of the septic tanks, the construction team found human bones. One of them was a perfectly preserved skull, so there was no denying what we were looking at, and I had a sinking feeling that it would cause problems for the team.

I called the Aceh police, like an idiot, to tell them we had found bones. They said, 'Yes, there are a lot of bones around.' Thirty thousand people had disappeared during the tsunami and were never found, and there was no forensic testing in Aceh to identify bodies. There were no records to identify them with, anyway. One of my team members had lived near the site; he explained that many bodies had floated down the river, building up in the estuaries and blocking the flow of water. He and others had pulled bodies out of the water and buried them on the nearby banks. This is likely what we had found.

The police advised me to call the local imam. We dug up the remains and put them in a large cardboard box, and the imam came to say a few words and carry the remains away. I assumed that would be the end of it, but things escalated very quickly. I got a call on Saturday to advise that a carpenter had gone crazy and jumped from the roof of a house he was working on, sliding down a river embankment that was encrusted with oysters and mussels. His legs and back had been sliced to ribbons by the shells and he was now in hospital in a semi-catatonic state.

The local team was completely freaked out; they didn't want to go back to work. They were all very clear that the man was possessed and the spirits didn't want us on the site. Even the Maori team leader was shaken; he told me something had come to him during the night and blown freezing air in his ear, and other reports were coming in from the team that spooky things were afoot.

'Right, how do you normally deal with this type of issue?' I asked. *How do we take care of the ghost situation?*

The team advised me to get the imam back in to do a spiritual cleansing and, to everyone's surprise, I agreed. I'd seen my fair share of traditional healers and cultural magic by then and I recognised that working with them was just part of the job. It's not that I believe in ghosts, but the team did, which created a problem for me. It had to be resolved in a way that would keep the team happy, so we brought the imam back in.

Interestingly, when we told the guy in hospital that we were going to do a cleansing, his eyes stopped rolling back in his head, he started to communicate with us clearly and his health rapidly got better.

The imam came on a quiet Sunday afternoon and walked the whole length of the site, muttering prayers. He paused near a site where we wanted to build a playground, then later at the place where we had found the bones. He then gathered the labourers together in a circle and started chanting, and they began to chant along with him. The imam was chewing a bright green substance that stained his lips. As the prayers continued, he walked around the circle, rubbing goo from his mouth behind the ears of each man. I was standing at a polite distance, watching, but the hairs on the back of my neck were standing on end.

At the conclusion of the ceremony, everyone seemed relieved. The imam told us that the ghosts had accepted that we had no other land and they would allow the villagers to stay, but we had to make a couple of changes to accommodate their burial places. One of the houses would have to be moved a metre to the left and the playground needed to be somewhere else altogether, but otherwise we were sweet. Everyone was happy. We had two more camp sites allocated by then and I suggested we cleanse them before we started. 'You know . . . just in case.'

The team had been very uncertain about working for a woman, but the whole incident seemed to boost their faith in me and bring everyone together, and the project moved at a cracking rate after that.

When the imam's bill came in, it was astronomical: 8 million rupiah, roughly A$800. I asked him for a receipt but he didn't deal in receipts, unfortunately, so I had to write my own. A couple of weeks later, I got a call from Red Cross headquarters to let me know that the receipt had been rejected.

'What?' I asked. 'Why?!'

'Amanda, you've sent us a receipt for *ghostbusting*.'

'Sorry, I didn't know what else to call it.'

When the river camp was finished, it looked fantastic. Two rows of houses faced each other across the access road we had built, sharing the water points and toilets that were installed every 50 metres. The community members took great pride in painting their houses and arranging pot plants on their porches, but within a couple of weeks they were complaining about the water. People were having trouble with their skin and had somehow decided that the water was bad.

I might never have figured out what the problem was if my co-worker hadn't fallen ill. I had had to leave Aceh briefly to have my appendix out and she had helped move the camp while I was away. She was diagnosed with typhus, a disease carried by lice, which made me re-evaluate the water problem. I went from house to house in the new settlement, examining people's skin, and sure enough they all had a telltale rash that suggested a lice infestation.

Working backwards, we realised that when the community had been moved from their old tent city to the transitional shelter site, all of their belongings had been packed into the one truck. The lice infestation had ripped through the site, carrying typhus with it. More than half of the families in the camp were now infected. If you discovered an outbreak like this today, you'd take it to the humanitarian cluster meeting and plan a tactical response with the help of other agencies and services. Without a cluster to rely on, I had to figure it out by myself.

The resettlement project transformed into a medical response as I sourced and circulated the typhus medication through the community and coordinated the treatment plan. The villagers had to apply an ointment and leave it on for twenty-four hours, which was tricky when their religion required them to wash every time they prayed, and to pray five times a day. Cut was my lead negotiator on all Islamic matters; she managed to convince people to let the treatment run its course.

All the clothes and bedding had to be boiled as well, so we bought a collection of forty-gallon drums, cut them in half and set them up at regular intervals along the road—massive boiling pots for a massive lice treatment. Everyone in the community would boil their clothes and leave them to dry in the sun. When the first load had dried, they would boil the clothes they were wearing.

We held meetings to explain the process to the women and they seemed to understand, but when the day came it was clear that the message hadn't gotten through. They hadn't started the coordinated process of sterilising their clothes. The pots were boiling but there was nothing in them, and the women were going about their usual routines. So we started over. I drew cartoons to explain the plan to the community, a comic strip showing the process step-by-step and hour-by-hour, and we went door-to-door in the village distributing copies. The next morning, before we even arrived on site, the community had mobilised. With the help of my little comic strip, they had the whole process under control.

As I might have mentioned, I'm quite tall. People in Aceh tend to be short and petite, and they were obsessed with the sheer size of me, which drove me insane. It got to the point where I couldn't go to the supermarket without getting papped. People would hide at the end of the aisle with their mobile phones and take sneaky photos of me as I walked past. I was usually dressed in construction gear and covered in mud from the building site, which was highly unusual for a woman in Banda Aceh. I started to get very self-conscious. In the end, I paid the housekeeper to do the shopping and avoided the supermarket altogether. The only time I went to the market was to buy the Sunday roast lamb.

During the week, I ate with my team. The Red Cross had had trouble finding a project manager to replace me and after the first two camps were successfully completed, they just stopped looking. I decided that the whole construction thing wasn't so hard, and when the projects got bigger I just increased the size of my team. I ended up with three local engineers, a health coordinator and an administration assistant—all young, but very dedicated. They were also very protective of me, especially when it came to food.

I was as timid as a little kid, eating the same nasi goreng or fried chicken dish for lunch every day, struggling with the heavy load of chilli that went into every dish. I realised that if I ate very quickly, I could push through the pain, and I drank a couple of glasses of lemonade with every meal to help wash it down. Once my team figured out what was going on, they were horrified. They started ordering for me every day and taste-testing my meal when it arrived. They asked for no chilli but there was always chilli in the food in Aceh, it was just about how much.

'No, this is too hot for you Amanda! Send it back!'

'Maybe this one?'

'Okay, this one is okay.'

As the construction projects got bigger, we brought caterers in to make lunch for the team. They'd cook for me too, but it was generally plain rice, since that was about all I could handle.

I was working six days a week in Aceh because the projects were intense, but Sundays were mine. On Sundays, I'd fire up the

Weber at the Red Cross house and put my roast on to cook, then head to the beach with the Red Cross team for a swim. By the time we got back and cracked our beers, the lamb would be just about ready.

Sunday roast was a steady tradition for nearly the whole year I was in Aceh, but we visited the beach less often as time went along. The coastline changed nearly every time we were there. There were strong rips, then there weren't; the shoreline would be shallow and long, but the next week it would drop away. Once, I went to dive through a wave and struck a *mandi* underwater—thankfully my hands collided with it before my skull did. Another day, I stood in the water and felt chunks of coral underfoot that were too smooth. *It's not coral, it's bones*, I thought with horror. Maybe it was, maybe it wasn't; I couldn't shake the feeling either way. The whole coast was a graveyard. And the beautiful ocean where we hung out and swam had unleashed that tidal wave of death.

There were so many young kids in the camps and they had lost so much; they needed a place where they could just be kids again. They needed space between the rubble and the construction, and the constant reminders of the tsunami. This is why we wanted to build playgrounds in the camps—they would help the little people heal.

Playgrounds in Indonesia were made of cement and iron bars, which horrified me as a nurse—too many potential broken bones. Thankfully, I found an alternative in a Thai hardware store: a giant plastic playground set that could be shipped in pieces to Aceh. Unfortunately, it didn't come with instructions. We had a colour photograph of the finished product and we had to figure it out from there. I spent several weekends on site screwing swings and jungle bars together.

The community from the sawmill had touched my heart a little bit, so I bought them a particularly large playground set. It had a spiral slippery dip and the local labourers did their best to assemble it without me, but things went awry somewhere, so they started to improvise. They brought in some extra materials to prop the whole thing up, and the slippery dip ended about a metre and a half above the ground. I realised they'd never actually seen a playground set before.

A baby was born shortly afterwards in the same camp, one of the first babies conceived after the tsunami. The community was very concerned for her. They told me she couldn't go to the toilet. I went round to take a look and very quickly found out why. The little girl had been born with a severe birth defect; she didn't have an anus. There was a tiny hole, but no sphincter, and the baby was starting to get irritable. She would get very sick in the near future if we didn't do something to help.

We took the baby to the hospital in Banda Aceh and were glad to learn that the internal organs were normal. The surgical team could fix the external issue, but there would be a significant cost to the family. It obviously wasn't going to happen unless the Red Cross paid for it. Mindful of the recent ghostbusting drama, I didn't know if I could get away with an invoice for a new anus, so rather than try to pay for it out of the company coffers, I decided to hold a fundraising barbecue. We held parties with the other Red Cross teams regularly, why not hold one for a good cause? I sent an invitation around. It said, 'Don't be an arsehole. Buy an arsehole.'

We ended up raising three or four hundred dollars, which was more than we needed for the baby's bottom. We considered throwing ourselves a self-congratulatory party, but decided that the extra money should go to a man who begged at the traffic lights near the Red Cross house every day. He had a severe facial deformity: an elongated nose that looked like an elephant's trunk. Over a few Bintang beers, we decided we'd send him to the hospital for an assessment and then throw another barbecue fundraiser and raise whatever further funds were needed to fix his face. We were feeling very charitable and proud of ourselves, but the man with the deformity told us to bugger off.

'My face is my livelihood!' he told us. 'If you fix it, I'll have to get a job.'

It was probably for the best. As a general rule, we knew it wasn't a good idea to raise money for specific individuals when you were in-country on an aid mission because it created unrealistic expectations in the community. It could also cause security issues if there were misunderstandings around money. But sometimes it just seemed counter-productive not to help the people you'd been sent to help.

By mid-2006 I had completed three transitional camps and my work in Aceh was beginning to wind down. I made it to Simeulue, finally, though not as a health promoter. They were now flying me around the country to consult on building projects, which I thought was kind of funny. A transitional camp built on the island kept flooding in heavy rains, because it had been built on top of a rice paddy without proper ground preparation. The whole thing became a wet sock in bad weather.

While I was dealing with this, I was asked to attend a media event hosted by the governor of Banda Aceh. The governor had given us the land where the other transitional sites were built, and the press conference, as far as I knew, was to celebrate the success of our program. The Australian Red Cross had moved many hundreds of people out of tents and into transitional housing—a big win for all. My job was to stand next to the governor and smile while he praised our work.

The press conference was held in the carpark of an abandoned football stadium, near to where the first long-houses had been built. I didn't get much of what was going on as everyone was speaking Indonesian, but I smiled and nodded on cue. The governor said my name, I smiled and nodded. The governor said the words 'Red Cross', I smiled and nodded again. Smile and nod, smile and nod. I thought it was going well. Then I realised that my translator, Ivan, was looking a little frantic. He was gesturing wildly from the crowd. Something was clearly wrong, but there wasn't much I could do about it while we were on live television.

When the broadcast ended, the governor reached over to shake my hand. 'Thank you so much, Amanda,' he said. 'I am very pleased that you will be moving the TV camp.'

'I'm sorry, sir?' I replied dumbly.

'We will discuss the details tomorrow,' he said.

The governor walked away looking very pleased and Ivan ran over to explain what had happened. On camera, the governor had asked the Australian Red Cross to build transitional housing for the last camp in Banda Aceh, for a community that was still living in tents on the grounds of Aceh's TV station. The site for the transitional camp was the abandoned football stadium behind us. I had about six weeks until the end of my contract to move more than a thousand people there. I had just smiled and nodded my way into a major housing project.

'Can you do it?' my boss asked.

'I'd need tons more staff, our team isn't big enough . . .'

'Can you do it?'

'It'll cost thousands and thousands to get it done in that timeframe . . .'

'Yeah, but can you do it?' she asked.

'I can do anything,' I replied.

'Right, just get it done.'

There were some complications with the TV camp, which complicated our planning. We heard rumours that the camp included many empty tents, which were only occupied when other aid organisations came around to make beneficiary lists for permanent housing. Text messages would circulate and people who already had housing would turn up to get their name put on a list, ensuring that two or three new houses were built in their name. I was unsure if we actually needed the football stadium camp, or how big it should be, but the governor was married to the project so he took care of the problem. The military turned up to the TV station camp in the middle of the night and blocked all the entrances, then went tent to tent counting heads to figure out who was actually living there.

We ended up with 400 families. We had to build 400 transitional shelters, which was more than I had built at the other three camps combined, and in about a quarter of the time. Still, I was really excited about the project. The other camps I had built were limited by the awkward shape and position of the land we were allocated. With the land available at the football stadium, I could build a textbook settlement, using all the lessons learned from the previous projects.

Traditionally, refugee camps are built in hard, straight lines to maximise the use of space. That's what we're used to seeing on TV—rows and rows of pale brown tents, stretching off into the horizon, all facing the same direction. But the ideal design for a displaced persons' camp is actually neighbourhood blocks, with clusters of houses sharing a big backyard space. The community could organise itself around the shared outdoor spaces—I was going to build gardens and clotheslines there—and because all of the houses were connected, domestic violence became a community issue. When everyone shared a communal backyard, the women felt much safer.

The project was a monster. My workforce swelled to 400 local people and sixty tradesmen. The ground in the stadium was flat, at least, but we had to build access roads, an electricity grid and a massive septic and water distribution system. I learned to do engineering calculations for weight-bearing roads and extended my knowledge of physics when it came to water pressure, and I became quite obsessed with urban design factors. It turned out that the spare ground we had to leave for septic system run-off was actually a safe and practical place to plant certain vegetables, which meant we had food-producing gardens between each of the houses. We built a mosque and a clinic on the site, and a large community playground, built to Australian standards, which I found on an Australian playground standards website.

We didn't have time to paint the buildings, but it had to be done to seal the wood. So I bought paint in a range of colours and asked the community members to come and choose the one they wanted, then use it to paint their own house. They saw it as a huge contribution to their struggle for dignity and a way to take ownership over their own homes; I saw it as a week's reduction in construction work. I was literally racing against the clock to get the camp done before my contract ended, and the whole team was racing alongside me. We had T-shirts printed: they had a Red Cross logo on the front and a picture of Bob the Builder on the back along with the slogan 'Yes we can!'

There were TV crews filming when we moved the community into the football stadium. These were the last displaced people in

Banda Aceh to be moved out of tents, so it was an important day for the whole region, a sign that vital progress was happening. I got a huge amount of kudos for the work, which was flattering, although I knew that it was at least partly because the camp looked great in pictures. There were plenty of important programs in Aceh that weren't quite as easy to photograph.

Still, I was proud of what we had achieved. The Clinton Foundation ran an assessment of the transitional shelter projects in Banda Aceh and our camps were highly commended, particularly the football stadium, because it was more than just shelter; it was designed to the health and wellbeing of the community. I was looking at everything from a public health perspective, and that made all the difference. It wasn't just a matter of putting a roof over people's heads, it was about keeping them free from disease and danger, and helping to preserve their dignity so that they could claw back from the trauma they had experienced.

The settlements we designed weren't cheap. The engineers working on similar projects for other aid organisations were thinking about speed and cost. I spent nearly A$1.6 million in six months, but that's what the money was for. We couldn't spend it fast enough. And while mine were the most expensive camps, they were also the most humane. In the best-case scenario, we'd do it that way every time.

After twelve months in Aceh, I had quite a broad skill set. I was a qualified nurse with three-quarters of a Master of Public Health degree. I could also drill boreholes and build refugees camps, but I wasn't technically qualified for the work. I figured I should get a piece of paper that said I was, so I enrolled in a Water and Sanitation in Emergencies course at the University of Copenhagen and spent the next month studying alongside engineers, learning the proper physics calculations for water pipelines and other basic maths. The final test included a lot of public health questions, so I had an advantage, but I turned out to be quite good at the maths as well. For the final assessment, we had to design a refugee camp. I finished at the top of my class.

# 7

# THAT LID LOOKS SHARP

I hadn't worked as a 'real' nurse for well over twelve months, so I thought I would try to refresh my skills while finishing my master's degree. I registered with a nursing agency and took bits and pieces of remote nursing work, including a stint on the Torres Strait Islands and another on Cape York. During this time, I was also sent to a tiny clinic in the Northern Territory—a place called Ampilatwatja, just over 300 kilometres north-east of Alice Springs.

There was a new nurse working there on his first remote gig, an ex-police officer called Liam. He was doing a great job, by all accounts, but he was struggling with the female patients due to cultural sensitivities in the community. The women didn't want to see him. The health service wanted a woman out there to manage regular consultations with women in the community and to provide some basic maternity support. More than anything, I was excited to see the desert again. I hadn't been back out there since I left Alice Springs.

The population of Ampilatwatja was no more than 400 people; it was a tiny community clustered around a red dirt football field, an airstrip and a small community shop. Surprisingly, the nurses' accommodation was more than comfortable. I had a nice little studio apartment built out of corrugated iron and curved just like an aircraft hangar; it was the only place I could escape from the crippling desert heat. It was the middle of summer and temperatures were well over 40 degrees on most days. I didn't do much but work at the clinic and sit in my apartment playing PlayStation, doing my best to avoid the study that I was meant to be finishing.

I wasn't around long enough for this routine to get boring. I also didn't have much time to get to know the community very well, although one thing did make an impression. Ampilatwatja was full of mad Brisbane Lions fans and every child under the age of five had been given the last name of a Lions player. I wanted to get all the 'Lions' kids together and take a photo to send to the club. Maybe the community would get a few free footies out of it.

Unlike Aurukun, Ampilatwatja was a dry community, so the alcohol-related problems didn't really exist. The clinic was busy during the day, but I was rarely called in after hours. I went a whole first week without a call-out, but things ramped up on the first Friday evening, when a man came in after having a convulsion. He needed to be evacuated, so I had to stay with him until the Flying Doctors arrived. I was still in the clinic when Liam arrived for his shift the following morning, which meant I was due for a ten-hour break, so I went back to my apartment to sleep. Within an hour, the phone rang and Liam was on the other end of the line. He wanted to know if I had driven the ambulance home, which I had. 'Good, just keep it,' he said. Michael, our janitor, had asked if he could take the vehicle to go kangaroo hunting, but Liam had refused him.

The clinic in Ampilatwatja was run by the local Aboriginal council, not the state government ministry of health, as the

Aurukun clinic had been. The council managed the funds for the health service in the way that best suited the community, and it meant that the community had more ownership of the clinic. No one would have even thought to ask to use one of our ambulances in Aurukun—they were official government vehicles—but apparently in Ampilatwatja it wasn't uncommon for a local to want to commandeer a LandCruiser. Politically, it was kind of tricky, and no one had bothered to brief us. It didn't take me long to realise that the clinic was managed very differently to Aurukun or even the clinic I'd worked at in the Torres Strait Islands. There were no Aboriginal health workers in town and neither Liam nor I understood how the system worked, which turned out to be a problem.

Liam called back a little later and told me Michael had left with the other car that belonged to the clinic. He asked if I could bring the ambulance back over so that he had something at hand in case of an emergency. 'No problem,' I told him. I was just up the street.

Oddly, when I walked outside, I ran straight into Michael, who lived across the street from my apartment. He was standing in front of his house eating a can of Spam. He had peeled back half the lid, squeezed half the meat out of the can and was eating it like an apple. *That lid looks sharp*, I thought, *that doesn't look safe*.

'Hey Michael, what are you doing with the car?' I said. 'Liam is looking for you—' As the words came out of my mouth, Michael threw the can of Spam at my head.

It was like one of those scenes from *The Matrix*. The meat stayed inside the tin, but I could see it spinning through the air, flipping over and over in slow motion, the razor-sharp edges of the jiggered can whizzing past my head. I managed to step out of its path and turned to see it explode as it hit the ground. In that moment of distraction, Michael had stumbled angrily towards me and I realised he was severely intoxicated. *Fuck*. I had played this wrong.

Michael grabbed the front of my shirt and I tried to be very passive, putting my hands up in the air as he growled in my face, his chest bare and his jeans falling down over his skinny hips. I danced backwards to avoid him as I tried to think of a way out of the mess I was in. Luckily, Liam had come out of the clinic and had seen what was happening down the street, and had raced over. As Liam approached, Michael let me go and I managed to put a bit of distance between us, but Michael continued swearing and raging, so both Liam and I had to retreat. We stumbled backwards towards the clinic. We needed to get inside.

People came out of their houses to watch. If something like this had happened in Aurukun, someone from the community would have stepped in, but Liam and I were both relatively new in town, so all we had was spectators. I managed to get the keys out and was trying to unlock the heavy clinic door before Michael reached us, but I was too slow. Michael grabbed Liam, lifted him off the ground and smashed him against the wall, splitting the back of his head open. The door swung open and I reached to pull Liam away from Michael, but there was no room. Michael was incredibly aggressive. I couldn't get between them and I honestly didn't think we were going to make it inside.

Then, out of nowhere, Michael's wife turned up with a huge nulla nulla stick and cracked Michael over the back of the skull. He dropped Liam and we both fell through the door, closing it behind us.

We sat on the floor, backs against the door. Michael was still yelling on the other side, but the volume had begun to fade. 'You okay?' I asked Liam.

'I think so,' he said. He touched the back of his head; there were traces of blood on his fingers.

When the noise faded completely, I let out a huge sigh. 'I think Michael might be drunk,' I said.

Liam grinned. 'Uh yeah, you think?'

We both laughed, but the confrontation wasn't over.

'Ya fuckin' white cunts, I'm gonna fuckin' kill ya!'

Michael was back and he still wasn't happy. I got on my knees, peeked through the window and saw him pacing up and down in the middle of the street with a shotgun in his hand. 'Ya fuckin' white cunts,' he screamed again. I looked down at Liam, who was still leaning against the door, assessing the damage to the back of his head.

'Does Michael have the keys to the clinic?' I asked. We both clicked at the same time. Michael was our cleaner; of course he had keys. 'The pharmacy?' I suggested.

The pharmacy was the one room in the clinic that Michael didn't have a key for, because it was where we kept the drugs. Liam and I scrambled along the floor and into the pharmacy, locking the door behind us. 'At least it's air-conditioned in here,' I noted, trying to lighten the mood a bit. Liam looked past me, nodding towards the door, which had a huge glass panel in the middle of it. It wasn't the best hiding spot.

We needed to call for help. There was nothing in the pharmacy to patch up Liam's head, which was still bleeding. I decided to leave the room for bandages and while I was outside dialled 000. There were no police in Ampilatwatja; the nearest police station was in Alice Springs, ten hours' drive away, but it was our best bet under the circumstances.

I realised I'd never actually dialled 000 before, and for some reason I got very nervous about it and tried to pretend it wasn't a big deal. 'Hi,' I said nonchalantly, 'my name is Amanda, I'm a remote area nurse in Ampilatwatja, and we're having a little situation.' I explained what was going on and the operator wanted to know if there was an ongoing threat to our safety. I looked out the window. Michael was still pacing around outside, cursing our names and waving his gun in the air. The wound on Liam's head was bleeding steadily. 'Uh, yes,' I replied.

'Okay, we have a team on the Sandover Highway. Sit tight, they should be there in about four hours.'

'Right, thank you,' I laughed. 'Tell my mum I love her, 'cause we're not going to last that long.'

The only other white person in town was an older guy who ran the local store; he'd been in Ampilatwatja for years. I hadn't met him but Liam had, and Liam seemed to think he was decent. We thought maybe we'd give him a call. At the very least we should warn him that Michael was on the rampage and, who knew, maybe he could help.

'No problem, I'll come down,' he told Liam.

'Come down and do what?' I asked in disbelief. 'There's a guy with a gun outside!'

But the shopkeeper did come down, and he got things under control very quickly. He hopped out of his car and had a few words to Michael, and then Michael climbed into the car with him and both of them took off.

We had no idea what was happening, but we decided to make a break for it. We locked the clinic, climbed over the back fence and made our sneaky way over to Liam's house, which was a few doors down from the clinic.

We had to sit there and do nothing. We couldn't even have a drink, because there was no booze in town, other than the stuff that was in Michael.

After about an hour, we got bored, so I jumped the fence and snuck back to my place to grab the PlayStation. We sat on the floor playing *Lara Croft: Tomb Raider*, wondering when it would be safe to go back outside. Shortly afterwards, the shopkeeper came knocking on Liam's door to let us know that everything had blown over. Michael had been hungry and the shop was closed for the weekend. We wouldn't let him take the ambulance to go kangaroo hunting, so all he had to eat was Spam. Classic hangry man, plus drunk and armed. After they had driven off, the shopkeeper had taken Michael to the shop and opened it up for him so that he could buy some food, and now everything was copasetic.

As the shopkeeper was sitting in Liam's lounge room explaining all this, Michael turned up on the doorstep. *Shit.* Liam and I didn't want to hide, exactly, we just preferred to stand out of sight behind a wall and let the shopkeeper answer the door.

'Is Liam here?' Michael asked.

'No, sorry, mate, Liam's not here,' the shopkeeper told him.

'I can't find Amanda, either,' Michael said.

'Yeah, they both had an emergency. They had to go out.'

'Ah no, I need the keys to the cold room,' Michael said. He called the pharmacy the cold room because it was air-conditioned. 'My wife hit me on the head and now I've got a real bad headache. I wanna sleep in that cold room for a few hours.'

It was pretty clear he had absolutely no memory of threatening us with a gun.

The police arrived a couple of hours later and we told them everything was fine.

'It's not fine,' they said. 'Michael attacked you, he assaulted Liam and he threatened both of you with a weapon, and that's not fine.'

'Yeah, but these things happen,' we said. 'It was just a misunderstanding.'

I think Liam was embarrassed because he was a former police officer but hadn't been able to control the situation. I was embarrassed because my initial approach to Michael had been very

118

cavalier. I didn't recognise the signs that he was drunk, and I felt like I had set him off. The police told us we had to leave town for our own safety but we pushed back—we were the only medical care around.

'You were under threat and the community didn't assist you in any way,' the police told us. 'We strongly advise you to leave.'

Liam called in to the health service management team in Alice Springs and they agreed with the police, so in the end we had to clear out. With us gone, the community in Ampilatwatja had no emergency healthcare at all. If anyone got sick, the nearest community clinic was in Utopia, about an hour's drive away.

The police stuck close by while we packed up our stuff and went to speak to the Aboriginal Council representatives to let them know the plan. Then, as we were making our way out of town, the police went to arrest Michael.

I was in Ampilatwatja just a handful of days and it was hardly a career highlight, but it was the last time I worked as a nurse in a remote Australian community. Later, we were asked to give statements about the trouble with Michael and then the story made its way into Northern Territory parliament discussions, so there was a bit more weight and attention around the incident. I was really nervous about how it would be seen. I felt like we had run away and left a few hundred people without services, but it wasn't really interpreted that way. The parliamentary discussion was about security risks for remote area nurses and the ongoing failure to provide proper support for people working in those environments.

The problem seemed uniquely Australian to me in some ways. The Red Cross would never have sent someone as inexperienced as Liam into the field by themselves, but remote nursing in

Australia adhered to a completely different set of standards than what I was used to overseas. There were no security briefings, no daily check-ins, and most importantly no mandatory debriefings after security incidents. Support services were offered for nurses and doctors who had bad experiences, but if you used them you carried the stigma of not being able to cope 'out bush'. To some extent, these incidents were seen as just another part of the job. That's just not the way it should be.

# 8

## GULLIVER IN THE LAND OF
## THE LITTLE PEOPLE

I seriously considered studying medicine. The thought had been bouncing around in the back of my head since my student nursing days, and when I finished up in Indonesia it came bouncing back again. Doctors were a critical resource in emergencies and I thought it would be useful to expand my medical knowledge. I wanted to understand more, to do more, to be more than just a nurse.

Before I went to study in Copenhagen, I went to Sri Lanka for a couple of weeks to take a course in infectious tropical diseases as part of my master's degree and that put an end to any ideas about medical school. There were two nurses in the course, while the rest were all doctors, and the doctors all wanted to be doing the work I had already done. They didn't speak very highly about medicine as a career. They wanted to be out in the field, working in disasters and development, and they were enrolled in the program to try to find a way into that world.

On reflection, I decided I probably didn't need to spend another six years studying. When it came to public health, as opposed to clinical medicine, there wasn't a big difference between doctors and nurses in the field. I was already on the right path. I didn't need to wander off.

When I returned to Australia, I took a short contract back in Aurukun, just four weeks, but I offered to stay and set up a hygiene promotion program. By then, I was looking at things differently. Healthcare wasn't just about patients but about the environment and how people interacted with it. If I could run a program on Cape York similar to the program I'd run in South Sudan, I could make a serious impact on scabies and gastroenteritis in the community, and all the knock-on effects of those diseases. I put a plan together for the director of nursing in Aurukun, and did a presentation for the staff outlining the benefits of going out into the community with a strategic public health plan. The team was really enthusiastic about it; they just didn't have the resources to make it a reality. They said great, go ahead, if I could do it on top of my fifty to sixty hours a week of regular nursing duties.

While I was weighing up their offer, I received a call from one of my lecturers in Copenhagen. He had recommended me for a contract in Nepal, a private consultancy with Concern World-wide looking at water and engineering installations in remote communities. He suggested I apply for it and gave me a daily rate, and the money was astronomical compared to what I was used to. I was genuinely torn. I would have liked to stay in Aurukun, I knew I could make a difference, but I wasn't up for the fight it would take to get the job done properly. And the contract I was offered was in Nepal! I'd never been there before. I decided that I was more than ready to head back overseas.

Concern Worldwide had installed gravity-fed water systems in the Nepalese highlands, in areas that were previously inaccessible to outsiders because of a civil war between the government and Maoist militant rebels. Working around the conflict, Concern had distributed materials to communities on the mountains, and the communities had built the water systems with guidance from local supervisors. The supervisors had taken photos of the projects, but that was really the only verification Concern had that the work had taken place. I was hired to go and check that everything was kosher and see what impact the project had made.

I had never travelled in central Asia before and I was amazed at how frenetic everything was. South Sudan was a dustbowl and Aceh was in ruins, but Kathmandu was a sprawling urban mass, every inch of ground taken over by buildings, cars and people. All of it was built on unstable ground, on a fault line, surrounded by mountains.

They put me up at a relatively fancy hotel, even posh by my recent standards, and I spent the first day acclimatising and watching expat families play in the pool. There were a lot of foreigners in town doing humanitarian work and they weren't living lives of deprivation—they had big cars, big houses, nannies and their families had a lot of casual lunches. Most of them worked for the United Nations—UNICEF or the UN's WHO, any acronym you could think of. I realised for the first time that there was a whole industry built up around humanitarian and development work, and it could be quite an indulgent lifestyle. I thought they were a bit soft, but I filed it away as a solid retirement plan.

When I met Shannon, the country director for Concern, she was very interested in my size. She was barely four feet tall.

'You look quite strong,' she observed in an extremely thick Irish accent. 'Are you good at walking? I'm going to adjust your terms of reference.'

My 'terms of reference' were the conditions and parameters for the job. Shannon had intended to send me to the low-lying, more accessible communities where the project had been rolled out, but she took one look at me and decided I'd make a good mountain climber. She wanted to know how I'd feel about hiking through Nepal for four weeks. I told her I felt great about it.

I was flown up to a place called Nepalgunj with an engineer from Kathmandu who was decidedly less enthusiastic about the plan than I was. For some reason I had assumed that Nepal would be cold, but Nepalgunj was stinking hot, a humid tropical jungle right on the border of India.

The local project manager was a British guy named Doug, who had grown up in Kenya and lived like a local in Nepal. His hair was crazy and he was as skinny as a rake, but he was the only male expat in Nepalgunj and he had quite a big fan club among the local ladies. He ran a food security and livelihoods project in the area which had taken two years to design—on the long side of normal, in my opinion, but Doug was having the time of his life up there.

Doug briefed me and Harry, the local engineer, then we were put in a car for a four-hour journey to the literal end of the road. From there, we hiked. They warned me not to travel with too much luggage because I'd be carrying it all on my back, but old habits die hard. My first-aid kit took up half the room in my bag. I had a couple of T-shirts and a list of villages that we were supposed to visit. I had no idea where any of them actually were.

The road ended at the foot of a long suspension bridge, and beyond that there were mountains. When we arrived, a tiny old woman was crossing the bridge with a 25-kilogram sack of grain on her back, secured with a strap of fabric tied across her bowed head. That was how women transported goods in Nepal.

Our head guide was one of the local Concern supervisors. As

we prepared to set off, I asked him how long it would be until we arrived at the first village on the list. 'Four days,' he replied. Walk in the park. Good thing I'd had nothing to do in Aurukun for four weeks but run up and down the airstrip.

The low-lying mountains were lush and green, and streams frequently crisscrossed our path, carrying water down from the snowy peaks. It was a totally different landscape for me, more fertile and agricultural than I had seen before, and the people we met as we wandered around had a unique character, too. They were very, very small, for one thing. Their faces were a deep, sunbaked brown, lined with hundreds of tiny wrinkles that collapsed together when they smiled. They were very friendly, but extremely poor; they were dressed in bright rags, but covered in dirt. The women wore bright beads around their necks and nose rings made of gold.

At the end of each day, we would arrive in a village and our guide would ask one of the locals if we could stay in their house. This was apparently completely normal, and in accordance with Nepalese custom. They would provide us with accommodation and food, but we couldn't give them money. We were their guests. We'd sit with their family over a meal and talk, our guides acting as translators. It really didn't feel like work to me, it felt like an amazing holiday.

The houses were a bit awkward, that was the only problem. They were made of mud, with terracotta roofs, and the doors were absurdly small. Between the first and second floors was a plank of wood with notches cut out at intervals, which is what the villagers used for stairs. These stairs were not designed for someone my size. It became a nightly challenge, wobbling my way up the plank to a bed that was too small for me, my host family looking on with genuine fear and horror.

The one time we stayed in a house that had a regular staircase,

I put my foot through a step. I felt like Gulliver in the land of the little people. I was on my way down, wearing my backpack, and the wooden tread snapped clean in half under me. I managed to catch myself before my leg went all the way through but I ended up with a terrible scratch and the poor host family was mortified.

The gravity-fed water systems were completely different from the boreholes I had been drilling. They were designed to trap and hold water that was flowing down from the higher altitudes, boxing a natural spring and connecting it via a series of pipes to a tap. The engineering was pretty simple, relatively speaking. The real work was in laying the pipes, which could run five or six kilometres from the spring down to the village, and the villagers did all that work themselves, digging trenches down the side of mountains.

When we arrived at one of the villages that had been part of the water project, we would gather the community together and I would ask a set of questions designed to evaluate the effects. The interview technique is called 'snowballing'—I would know which direction to head in depending on what the previous responses had been, which is how we came to realise that the project had had unintended outcomes.

Concern had launched the water project to improve the quality of the water for communities in the region. The idea was that families were using still or surface water that may have been contaminated, leading to health complications in children, including diarrhoea. The gravity-fed water systems would provide a cleaner source, and by installing a piped water source that brought water close to the houses, we had bought the community valuable time. The women had previously spent four to six hours a day collecting water, leaving the house before dawn to source it, then going out again in the afternoon. It meant that their children didn't eat until they returned quite late in the morning, then maybe once again in the late afternoon, which wasn't frequent enough for healthy growth. With a water point closer to home, the women were able to stay home and feed their children more often. The water project had a massive nutrition impact, rather than being about hygiene.

One of the most remote villages we visited was at the top of a mountain. It felt like the end of the world. We arrived late in the evening and I realised that it was actually quite cold. We'd walked up out of the jungle and into the Himalayas.

There was a little office in the village that the community had designated for management of the water system, and I noticed minutes from their last community meeting tacked up on the wall. This was what I had wanted to achieve with the communities in South Sudan, but we never quite hit that level of sophistication. The Nepalese villagers really got it, though. They took the project very seriously, which was amazing to see.

The local women gathered on a slate terrace overlooking the mountains for our focus group, appearing out of the mist that was rolling in as the sun went down. They were so very tiny they barely made it up to the level of my rib cage, and almost every one of them was wearing glasses. An NGO must have been up in that part of the world running an optometry project at some point, but it was clearly a very long time ago. The glasses were like the bottom of Coke bottles, and scratched so badly that I was positive there was no way they could see out.

Some of the villagers we met hadn't seen a white person in decades, because of the war. We weren't in a tourist area where they would encounter hikers or adventure sports travellers, so I must have been quite a strange figure to see on their doorstep.

But the Nepalese were incredibly open and friendly. They smiled those crinkly smiles quite often, and everywhere we went they showed us the most incredible hospitality.

After a couple of weeks of walking through the mountains, I thought I'd developed a bit of a rhythm. Our guides were still walking ahead, but they had less of a lead, and I only really struggled on a steep incline. One day, an elderly Nepalese woman trotted past me up a hill carrying a huge load of maize in a basket on her back. It was a little  embarrassing, but I kept trudging away. When the woman got to the top, she put her basket down. *Must need a rest*, I thought, but no. The old lady bustled back down the hill to my side and started pulling at my backpack. She wanted to carry it up the hill for me. 'I can do it! I can do it!' I laughed, but she wouldn't hear of it. She hoisted the bag on top of her head like it weighed absolutely nothing and virtually sprinted back up the hill. At the top, she put my bag on the ground, picked up the basket of maize, gave me a little wave and then disappeared.

We got up around six every morning and started walking. By nine o'clock, little stalls would appear by the side of the road and we would buy sweet tea and Nepalese doughnuts for breakfast, which would keep us going until late in the afternoon, when we would find our next meal. I started buying cucumbers from the stalls in the morning and snacking on them as we walked. They were easy to keep in the pockets of my backpack and the high water content staved off dehydration.

The further we travelled into the mountains, the fewer villages we came across and the less we saw the roadside stalls selling cucumbers and doughnuts. We walked ten hours a day, book-ended with breakfast and then dinner when we arrived, and in between I dealt with a grumbling stomach and just got on with things.

One day, our walk stretched out to twelve hours. We hadn't found anywhere to stop for a meal and we still had quite a way to go. We came around a hill and found ourselves next to a wide brown plain, a dry riverbed with a trickle of water running through it. There were a handful of houses nearby but the village was on the far side of the riverbed, built into the side of a mountain. There was no way I was going to make it that far, I decided. I was hungry and tired, and it was already dark.

One of our guides took off for a nearby house and came back to tell us, with some excitement, that there was a hotel right beside us. By hotel, he meant a house with a room available to rent. And as it turned out, the room wasn't available. The owner was on his way out—he was on his way up the mountain to a baby-naming ceremony—but he agreed to let us sleep in the storeroom where he kept his maize. He apologised that he couldn't cook for us, but he was already running late.

I pulled out my bedroll and made myself a glass of rehydration salts and ate a handful of trail mix for dinner. Our guides were headed over to the village where they thought they might find food, but I was too knackered to even think about joining them. 'If you find something, let me know,' I told them, climbing into my sleeping bag.

In the morning, we had a plan. The owner of the house where we were staying had a property two hours' walk up the mountain and we were headed there for breakfast. We were invited to the baby-naming ceremony, where there would be plenty of food. *Two hours? No problem*, I thought. It had been a good twenty-four hours since our last substantial meal, so what would another two hours matter?

The two-hour walk was actually four hours, by which time I was about to drop off the perch. To make matters worse, the family had been waiting for us, dressed in their Sunday best. We were now the guests of honour at the baby-naming ceremony. *At least there's plenty of food*, I thought. There were huge pots of rice on the fire. Unfortunately, I would have to wait a bit longer to eat because the family had invited me to take part in the ceremony. Strictly speaking, only men were supposed to participate, but I guess they figured I was my own special category.

I was ushered into a little hut where a group of men gathered around a smouldering fire, which filled the room with smoke. There was a tiny, tiny baby in one of the men's arms and the other men were pinning money to the little white singlet it wore. *Ah right, I'm here to contribute some money!* When my turn came, I pinned a note on the baby, too.

People were talking to me, but I had no idea what they were saying, all I could think was that I really needed to eat. Things got fuzzy. I emerged from the smoky hut and there were people dancing, a blur of noise. And the rice, still boiling in the pot, like a shimmering mirage. It was actually a really lovely party, but it was also a bit like torture.

Eventually I was invited to eat, but upstairs with the women. Going upstairs meant walking one of those planks in my hazy, famished state while carrying a plate of food. *I can do it, I can do it*, I thought, and do it I did, just barely. When I sat down to eat, my hand was shaking. A couple of seconds later, I passed out.

When I came to, the whole room was in a panic. The men helped me to my feet and led me into another room, gesturing for me to lie down on the bed. The bed was really just one and a half metres of rope net tied to some flimsy-looking tree trunks. 'I can't lie on that, I'm going to break it!' I told them, but the family insisted.

I did not feel great. I lay stiff as a board on the creaky ropes with my feet hanging over one end, listening to the poor family downstairs continue to freak out. They had very likely never met a white person before, then in comes Gulliver, dancing at their party and then dropping like a stone. Our head guide was freaking out, too—he thought he had killed me—but Harry had a plan. He was asking for a donkey. As had been explained to me over the preceding couple of weeks, nobody rode a donkey in that part of the world unless they were pregnant or a hundred years old. Donkeys were for carrying goods, not people. It was all the motivation I needed to roll off the bed and finish the bowl of rice that had been left beside me. Twenty minutes after that, I felt fine.

'I'm alright! I'm alright!' I told everyone as I emerged from the house, but the party was a little muted after that. I am sure that to this day the elders of the village enjoy telling the tale of the white giant who came and collapsed in the middle of a naming ceremony.

One of the most remote villages we visited also happened to be the most unhygienic I had ever seen. There was open defecation and urination in the streets, and the villagers were so grimy their skin was black. When I ran the focus group, it emerged that they were dirty because they only bathed properly once or twice a year. It was just too cold to bathe regularly that high up in the mountains. The water project had included the provision of toilets, which should have stopped people from using the whole village as a toilet, but the toilet structures provided were so solid that the villagers had used them to store food. It made sense when you thought about it: why would you use the best building in your village for defecation? We'd delivered the hardware, in terms of the water infrastructure, but the more remote areas I visited were in need of some more software: hygiene and nutrition education programs to help them make the most of what they had.

I loved working in health and hygiene promotion. It was fantastic to sit and work with communities on these simple but incredible programs that genuinely changed lives. But the job had a bit of a downside. Generally speaking, the places that need hygiene promotion programs the most are the places without any hygiene. In Nepal, it meant that I hiked for weeks without a proper shower or toilet. I ate once, sometimes twice a day and dropped about seven kilos. I also got some sort of fungal infection that was aggravated by the hike. After one particularly arduous walk, which went downhill for eight hours straight, both of my big toenails went black and later fell off. I like to tell that story to anyone who thinks that humanitarian work is glamorous.

In total, I spent a couple of months in Nepal, including a short stretch of time in Kathmandu. In the city, you couldn't avoid working on earthquake preparedness. It was integrated into all humanitarian aid planning in the country and was a good part of the work done out of the Concern head office. It was a small part of my role in Nepal, but it left a huge impression on me because everyone viewed the situation with mild anxiety. The Himalayas form a perfect circle around Kathmandu and the earth that the city is built on is like Play-Doh; layers and layers of run-off sediment roll and bounce off the mountains when an earthquake hits, creating multiple shockwaves on top of the original shake.

It wasn't a matter of *if* an earthquake would hit, but when. And with everything so tightly congested there, we knew the disaster response would be a nightmare. There were no parks and no football grounds where people could be housed when the buildings came down, and the buildings where lined up like dominoes, some centuries old. The casualties were going to be massive.

The modelling of the earthquake that would hit Kathmandu was on the scale of Hollywood disaster movies—every scenario seemed worse than the one before it. I told the head of country that I was going to quit humanitarian work and become a scuba diving instructor when it happened.

An earthquake did hit Kathmandu several years later, a 7.2 magnitude quake that killed nearly 9000 people and caused $10 billion worth of damage, but even that wasn't the one we were waiting for. That earthquake is still on the way.

# 9

# FIFTY KILOS OF BETEL NUT

In the Solomon Islands, the Weather Coast is called the Weather Coast because it is pummelled regularly by storms. It's on the southern side of an island called Guadalcanal and it takes four or five hours to get there by boat if you're coming from Honiara in the north. Boat is the only way to reach the Weather Coast because the middle of Guadalcanal is impassable mountains and dense rainforest, but the boat can only take you so far. Once you get within sight of the beach, you have to jump out and body surf through the break to shore. The Weather Coast water dumps too heavily on the rocky coast to allow for a safe beach landing.

After Nepal, the Australian Red Cross offered me a placement in the Solomon Islands giving technical advice to the National Society about its hygiene and sanitation program. I would be based in Honiara, but the job involved regular boat trips to the south side of the island followed by a three-hour hike into the jungle to reach Guadalcanal's most remote village communities. It was tough going and the nurses who had been in the role before me had struggled with it. The Red Cross offered the job to me

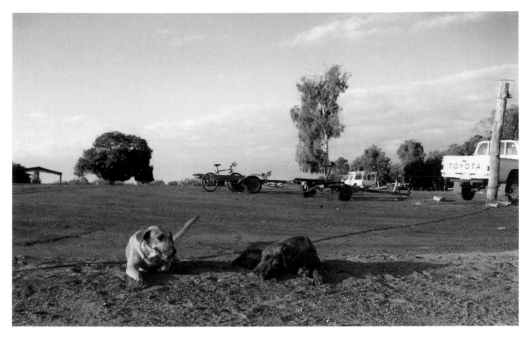

Three Rivers boat ramp with camp dogs. Aurukun, 2001.

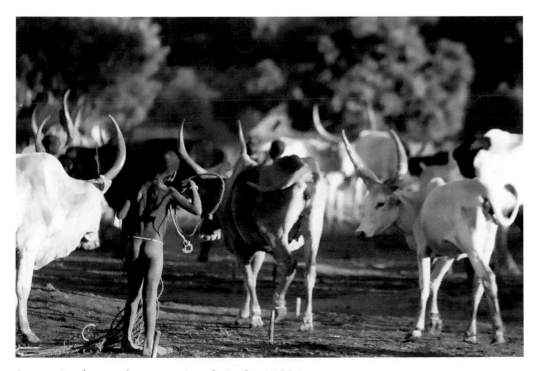

Sunset in the cattle camp, South Sudan, 2004.

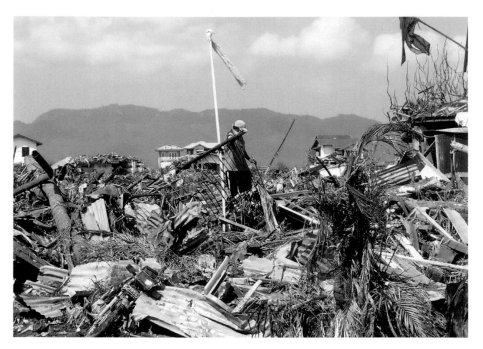

Banda Aceh, Indonesia, 2005. The level of destruction and clean-up still needed ten months after the impact of the tsunami.

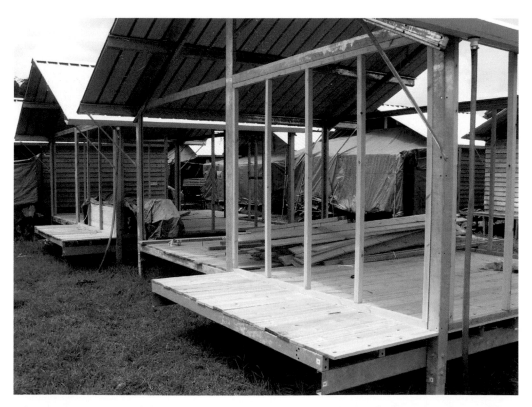

The construction of the transitional houses in Banda Aceh. Ten people could build one house in a day.

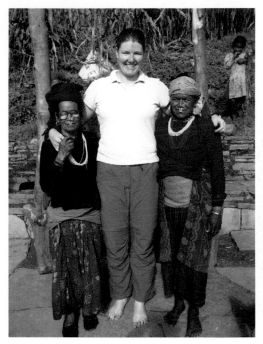

Meeting with the women's committee in the highlands of Nepal, 2007.

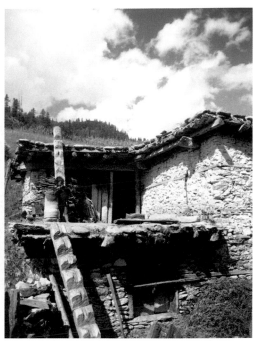

The precarious stairs, all over this part of Nepal.

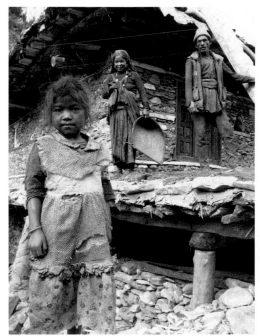

High in the Nepal mountains, where hygiene promotion was needed the most.

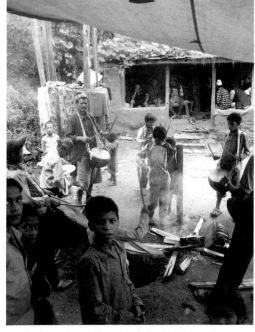

The baby-naming ceremony, where the townspeople are most likely still talking about the white woman who collapsed in their village.

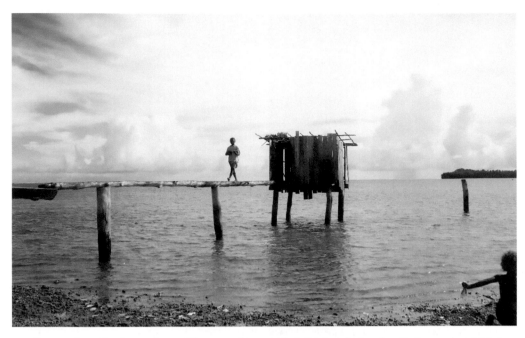

Walking the plank to the toilet on the artificial islands in the Solomons, 2006.

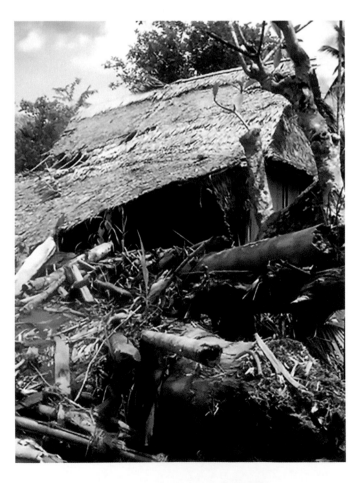

Damage caused by
Cyclone Guba in Oro
Bay, Papua New Guinea,
2007.

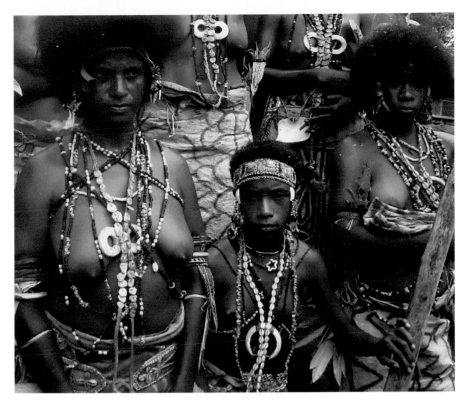

The welcoming committee in Oro Bay, just before I broke the house they built for me.

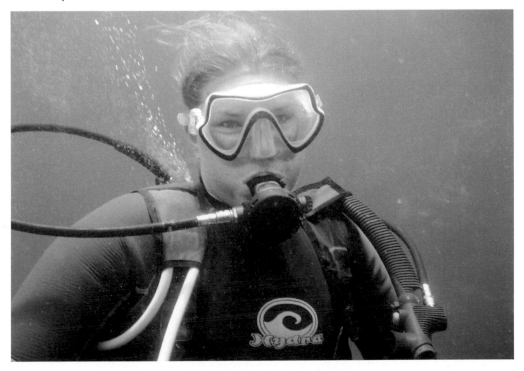

Time for a quick scuba dive in Oro Bay. It was amazing.

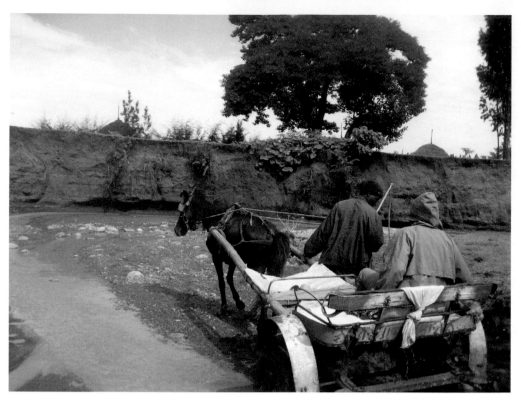

Delivering supplies via horse and cart in Shashogo, Ethiopia, 2007.

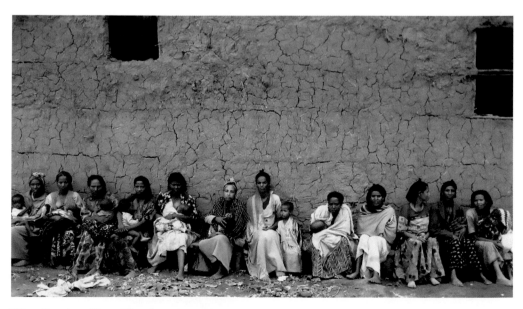

Distribution line, Shashogo.

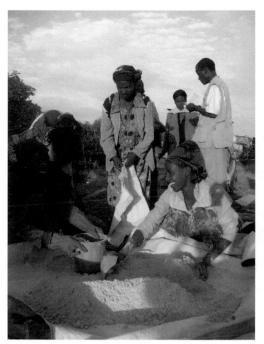

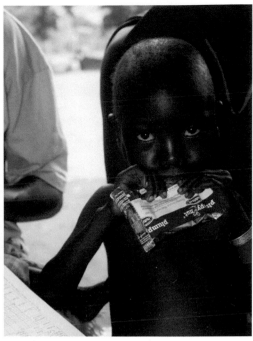

Mixing corn soya blend for moderate malnutrition late into the day in Shashogo.

Plumpy'Nut distribution in Karamoja, Uganda, 2008.

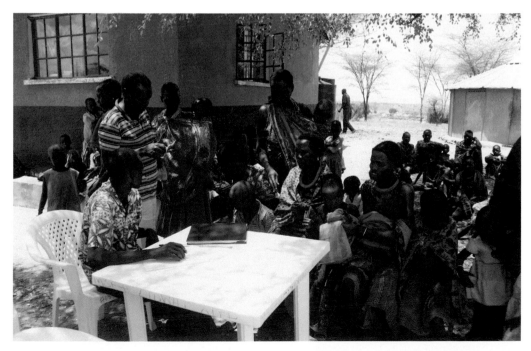

Discovering the prevalence of micronutrient deficiency in Karamoja led to mass screenings at all local clinics.

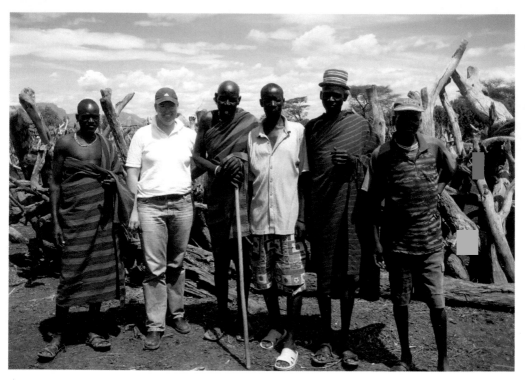

Meeting with village chiefs, Karamoja.

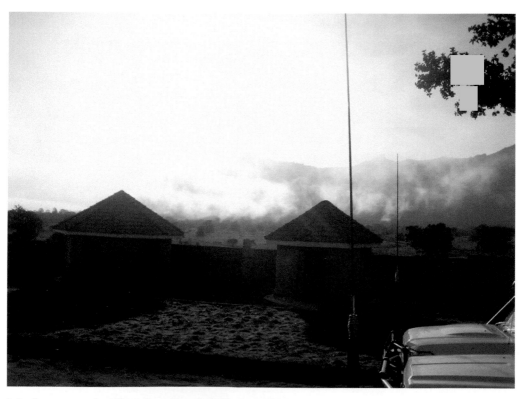

My home and office for six months in Karamoja.

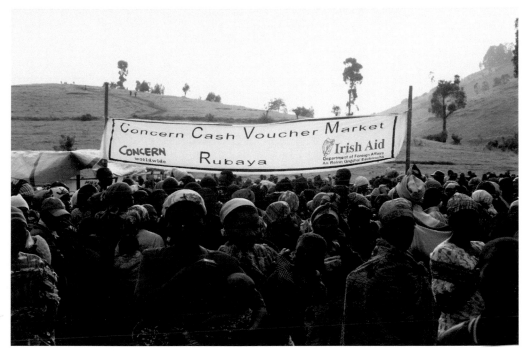

Day one of the voucher market in Rubaya, Democratic Republic of the Congo, 2009.

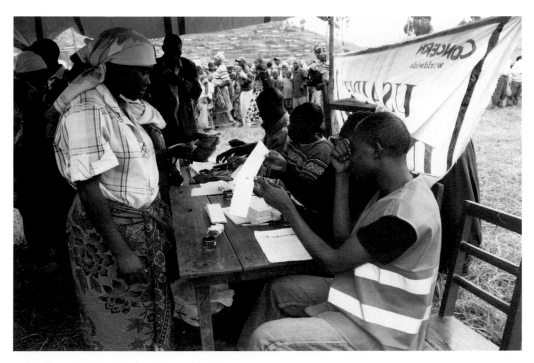

Voucher distribution point for the market in Rubaya.

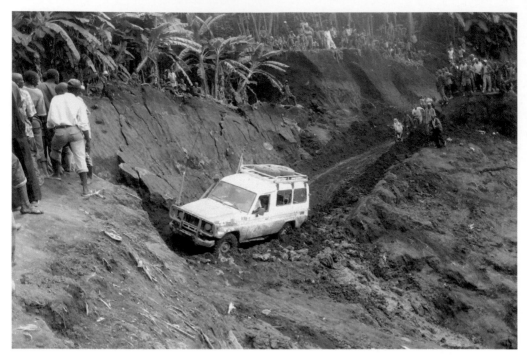

The muddy road to Rubaya. It became impassable a few days after this.

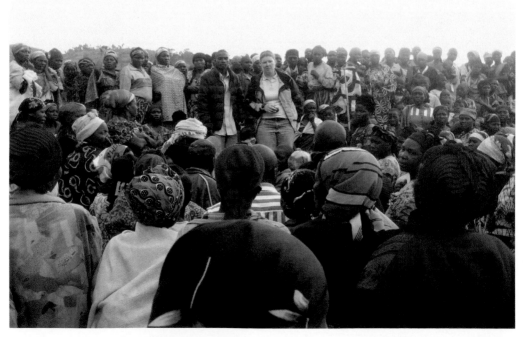

Informing the village that the voucher distribution would be postponed due to the arrival of Rwandan troops in the area, Rubaya.

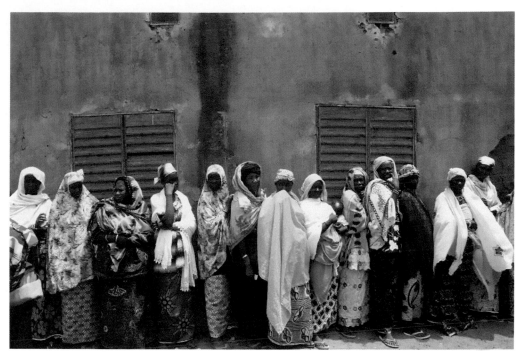

Cash distribution line in Tahoua, Niger, 2010.

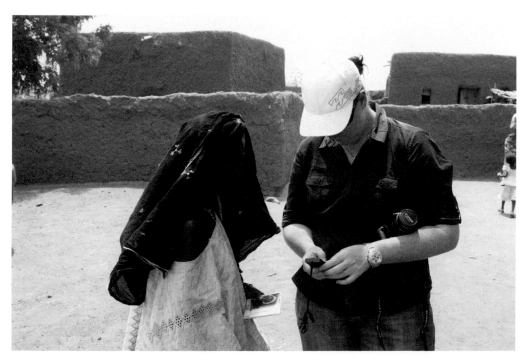

Cash distribution by mobile phone, Tahoua.

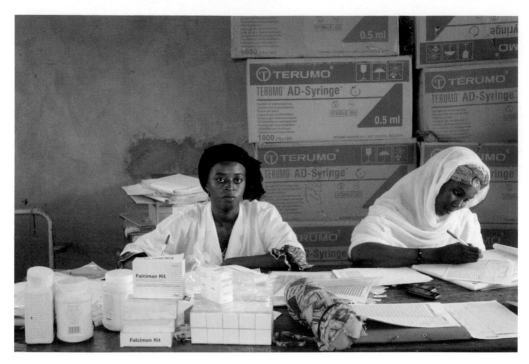

A clinic for malnourished children, Tahoua.

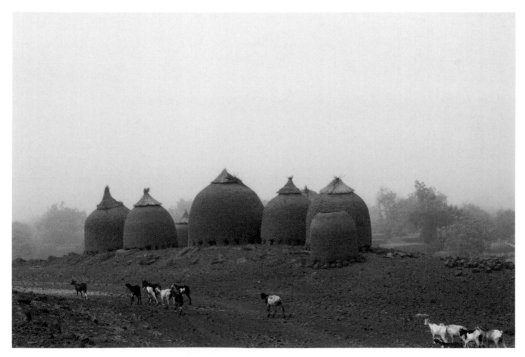

Grain stores, Tahoua.

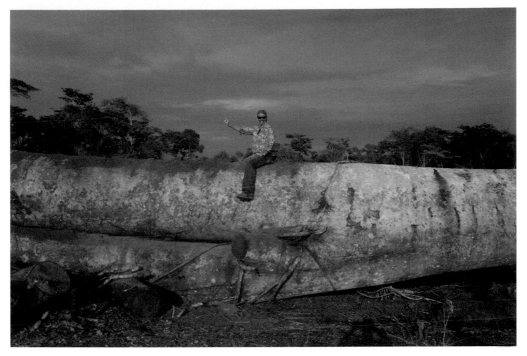

The middle forest tree, from the middle of the camp in Ziah, Liberia, 2011.
Almost a sudden end for me.

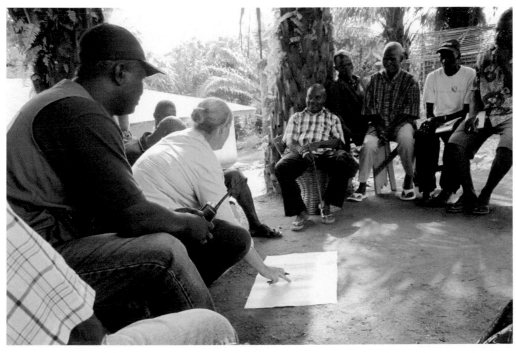

Planning the establishment of a more permanent camp in Ziah with the camp
committee.

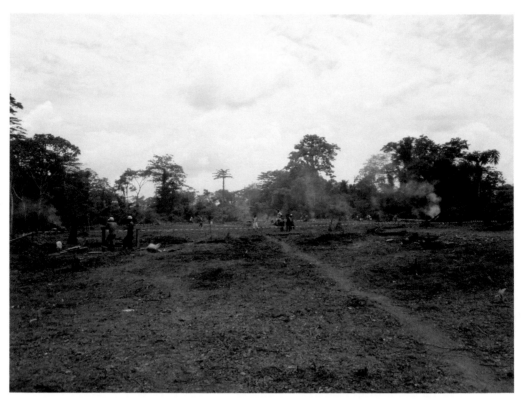

The camp in Ziah, before and after construction. Ten weeks. Three thousand people.

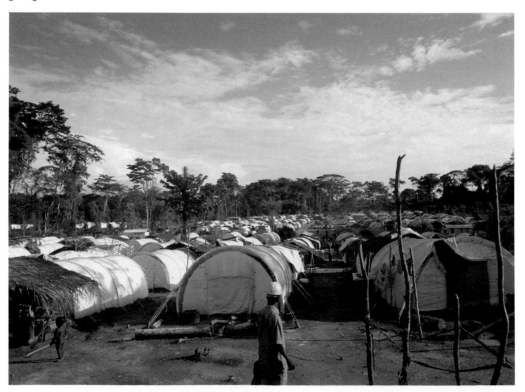

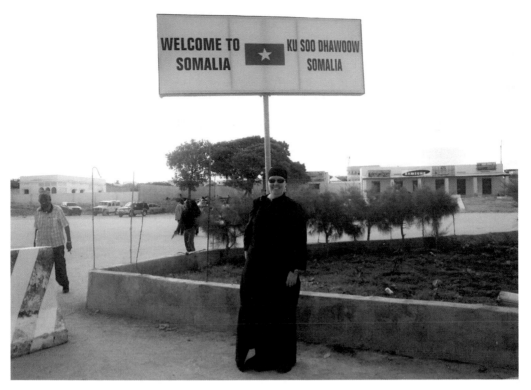

Mogadishu Airport, Somalia, 2011.

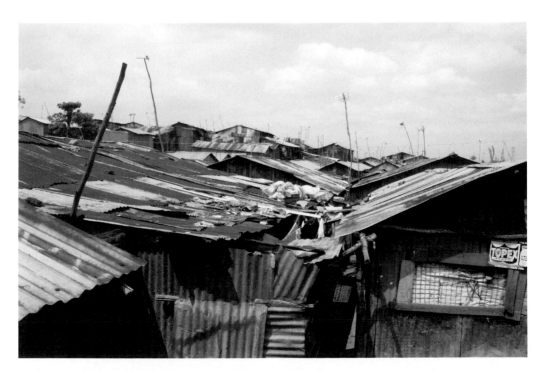

Urban malnutrition assessment in Kenya, 2011.

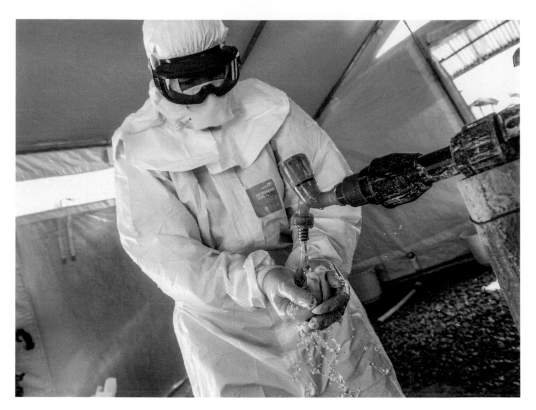

Leading the response at the Kenema Ebola treatment centre in Sierra Leone, 2014.
(Photos: Tommy Trenchard/Australian Red Cross)

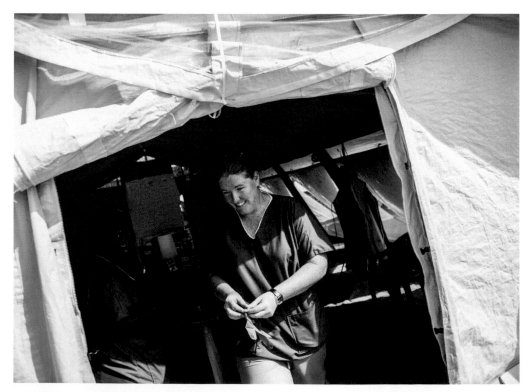

because it was more like camping than real work. They knew I'd think it was fun.

The Solomon Islands is an archipelago nation, a cluster of islands in the South Pacific, north-east of Australia, and it looks exactly like you'd imagine. The whole place is covered in coconut palms and fringed by white sand beaches which drift away into turquoise blue. People lead a very relaxed life out there and generally they're quite happy, but there were serious hygiene and nutrition challenges in the community which were largely dictated by poverty. Diabetes and obesity were rife, and people had limited access to decent healthcare. If disaster struck, they were also very vulnerable, with limited resources to help them recover.

I was sent down there on a capacity-building mission with the Solomon Islands Red Cross team, a little hand-holding by the Australian Red Cross to help strengthen and develop its work in at-risk communities. It was more teaching than doing, and it happened at Pacific pace: two or three hours of work a day, and a lot of waiting around in between. It was a very different speed than what I was accustomed to, but that was just the deal.

The Solomon Islanders had quite dark skin but their hair was bleached blonde or orange by the salt water and the sun. One of my team members had orange teeth, too, which came from chewing betel nut. He was a very relaxed cat. He was extremely tall, laughed all the time, and played the guitar well, which I had plenty of opportunity to experience when we were out in the field. The other local guy I worked with was short and stocky, also very laid-back; then there was the project manager. He was a bit older, in his sixties, but still very strong. Islander men are built that way— big and strong, though often overweight. When the men went out fishing, they would climb trees to collect coconuts, cutting their way through the jungle. Even among the most educated professionals, the culture was still very physical. Which was lucky, because the work my team was doing often took a bit of grunt.

The boat that carried us to the south side of the island was a large open dingy, about seven metres long. It was a very basic fibreglass vessel with three bench seats and a motor at one end, which made the ride around the coast both endless and uncomfortable. Getting supplies out of the boat was an art form. The two younger guys would swim to shore and the project manager, Ben, would stay in the boat, skating in and out on the wave, and hurling supplies towards the men on shore whenever he was close to the beach. When the boat was empty, Ben would steer it towards the shore, crashing it straight into the rocky sand so the other guys could drag it out of the water. It was incredibly tough going.

The hike into the jungle was intense, too. We had to wade across a river to get to one of the more remote villages, hoisting the bags and supplies over our heads to keep them dry. The field trip could last up to a week and we had to bring our own food supply as well as all the materials for the program. The villagers would share their accommodation with us, but we were responsible for our own dinner, except for pineapples, watermelons and coconuts, which were in abundance on the island and shared freely. There was no refrigeration out there and the food supply in the Honiara supermarkets was limited anyway, so we got by on two-minute noodles and Spam. The guys in my team were absolutely obsessed with Spam, and we were spoiled for choice; there was red can Spam and blue can Spam. The guys generally opted for the red can because it was a dollar cheaper, but after our first field trip I insisted on paying for the more expensive version. There was visible anatomy in the red can Spam. I'm pretty sure I ate an aorta.

Each family in the village communities I visited in the Solomon Islands had a small palm-fringed building to sleep in, but they lived most of their lives outdoors. They cooked, ate and rested outdoors, under a roof of palm trees, and only went inside at night when it was time to lie down. I ended up spending a lot of time inside the huts, on the other hand. The team from the Solomon Islands Red Cross spoke in local language to the villagers, and I didn't want everyone to feel as if they had to include me in their conversations. It was a very gentle, Pacific vibe; they all sit around playing guitar and singing together and the last thing I wanted to do was interrupt.

The community relied on rainwater for drinking, which was never in short supply on the Weather Coast, but for washing people used the river. The women bathed together, fully clothed in traditional skirts. The men would go down afterwards for their round, but they didn't really know what to do with me. In the end, I was given my own special bath time, and the villagers rang a church bell to let everyone know to steer clear when I was in the water. I didn't quite trust the system. I bathed with all my clothes on.

I read quite a few books during this relatively short contract, including Nelson Mandela's biography. The villagers were agrarians and they worked long hours on their crops. We had two hours' access to them each day to run the program, if we were lucky. The rest was just killing time. It was a lovely part of the world, but it could get a little boring, if I'm completely honest. I missed the intensity of the work in South Sudan and Aceh.

Naturally, there was no internet or television out in the jungle, just a faint radio signal for the VHF radio that was set up in the village. We called into the office in Honiara once a day, but it was just a safety check. We let them know we were okay, and they kept us up to date with the weather so that we could plan the best time to head back up the coast. On one particular day, head office told us to cut the program short and return immediately. There was a cyclone due to hit the island in a couple of days and we would be too exposed in the jungle. We had to bring the team back.

The team agreed to pack up before nightfall, get a decent bit of sleep and then head off before dawn so that we could reach the coast by sunrise—the early morning weather would be best for our boat trip back to Honiara. Ben woke me at 2 a.m. to tell me that the river was rising fast. While I was sleeping, they had been dealing with an emergency: some kids had been washed away while trying to cross the river, and the Red Cross guys had been paddling around in dug-out canoes, rescuing them. They woke me up to let me know that we could probably cross the river if we left immediately. If we waited, we'd miss the window and we'd be stuck there when the cyclone hit.

Our party was a little larger when we set out than when we'd arrived. One of the guys was bringing his pregnant girlfriend along, and she had brought a toddler. We were also carrying about fifty kilos of betel nut. Betel nut is a natural narcotic used in Asia and the Asia Pacific. It's an orange nut that's chewed for a mild, euphoric high. Betel nut was worth more in town than it was in the village, so the guys could sell it for a profit. They weren't inclined to leave that profit behind. So, in addition to the program gear and a couple of extra passengers, the guys were going to lug a few sacks of betel nut through the jungle. There was also a small piglet. Don't ask me why.

Several days earlier, when we had first crossed the river on foot, it had come up to the middle of my thigh. On the way out, it was as deep as my chest, and 30 metres wider on either side. The pregnant girlfriend was far too petite to navigate the river, so

I had to carry her under one arm. I used the other arm to balance my backpack on my head, but halfway across, Ben lost his footing and was nearly swept away. I dropped the bag to grab hold of him, but he managed to snag the bag and drag it along behind us. Somehow, I got all three of us (and the bag) safely across the river.

We made the three-hour trek from the river to the beach in the dark, in pouring rain, with sodden clothes and water-logged rucksacks. The sun was coming up just as we arrived, but we had no way of knowing what the cyclone was doing because we had no way of getting in touch with Honiara. We weren't travelling with a satellite phone. I should have known better, but I trusted the local team and they were very relaxed about the field trips to the Weather Coast; they made the journey at least once a month. I hadn't bothered to check safety or security procedures beyond basic radio checks.

The surf was monstrous but the last information we'd had was that there was a window of opportunity before the cyclone hit, so we decided to take it. There was no way we'd make it if we turned back to the village, anyway. It took quite a while to load up the cargo and crew, what with having to toss everything on board and the passengers having to swim out, but when we were finally ready to go, the ocean looked reasonably good. The water was flat, almost like a mirror. It was the sky overhead that was worrying.

We didn't make it very far along the coast before the guys cut the engine. 'What are you doing?' I asked.

'We need to put the fuel in the tank,' Ben explained.

They had a jerry can full of fuel but the motor was almost out, and there was no way to refuel while we were bobbing around at sea. 'Should we maybe have done that before we got into the middle of the ocean?' I asked. This was Islander logic for you.

The guys had to detach the fuel tank from the engine and swim it into shore, along with the spare fuel, to complete the operation. Meanwhile, they left me bobbing on the water in a motor-less boat with a pregnant woman, a toddler and a small pig. Needless to say, there was no anchor.

*We're on the edge of the Pacific,* I thought to myself. *There's nothing between us and South America.*

To the guys' credit, they seemed very relaxed about everything, and I liked to roll with the punches. They fuelled the tank, swam back and got us moving again. They were calm, so I was too. Then we rounded the corner of the island, and they were suddenly quite a bit less calm. Out in the channel, the ocean was heaving. And then it started to rain.

The boat was struggling against the waves, barely making headway. The front of the boat lurched into the air and slammed down with each wave, bouncing us up and down on to the fibre-glass bench seats. I thought my kidneys would start to bleed. The kid was wailing, as was the pig, and I started to do mental calculations. We were no more than about five hundred metres from the shore at any point and I knew I could make it. The question was, who would I take with me? The boys could obviously swim, so they could fend for themselves. Could I manage the pregnant woman and the toddler? Maybe. What about the pig? Probably not. Whatever happened, I was definitely leaving the fucking betel nut.

We'd been in the boat for six to seven hours and were still nowhere near Honiara. *This is bullshit! Surely there is a better plan?* I told the guys we needed to land wherever we could and build ourselves a shelter. I figured we must be close to running out of fuel. It was only a four-hour trip on the way out. They told me to hang on for just a little bit longer. A couple of beaches further along, we would reach the road that ran from the city down to the base of the island. If we landed there we could get word back to the office, and they could send a car for us.

Miraculously, we made it that far, beaching the boat on shore so that we wouldn't have to fight the surf and piling everyone out in the rain. There was a village in the cove where we took shelter and a phone in the village so that we could call back to the office in Honiara. They told us that the cyclone had hit early. We were right in the middle of it. They'd send a car, but it would take a couple of hours to reach us, so we might as well sit back and enjoy the storm.

There was a large international police force in the Solomons known as RAMSI, the regional assistance mission to the Solomon Islands. The Australian Federal Police force made up the large majority of the force along with some Kiwis and police from Papua New Guinea, Fiji and other Pacific nations. Despite the laid-back nature of the Solomons, it had experienced turbulent times, particularly when land disputes had spilled over in 2003. An Australian police officer had been ambushed and killed in 2005 and not long before I'd arrived rioting had occurred, with shops owned by foreigners burned and looted. Heavily armed police patrolled the streets of Honiara, in shorts and Teva sandals.

I shared my hotel in Honiara with a group of helicopter pilots who were in the Solomons servicing the armed forces. They were older blokes, ex-military. They told a lot of dad jokes, drank top-shelf spirits, and every one of them had a nickname. We used to joke that they had AIDS: Aviation Induced Divorce Syndrome. They were tough guys, but they all looked out for me.

When I finally got back to the hotel after the Weather Coast adventure, I had to walk through the dining room of the hotel soaking wet. It had been sixteen hours since the local team had woken me up and told me we had to get moving. I'd certainly looked better at the end of a work day. The pilots took one look at me and their mouths fell open. 'Where the fuck have you been?!' they asked. 'There was a cyclone.'

'Yeah, I am aware,' I laughed. I explained what had happened.

'Why didn't you call us? We would have come and picked you up in a chopper.'

The helicopter flight from Honiara to the Weather Coast takes about fifteen minutes because you go right over the top of the mountain. I couldn't have got in touch, but I wasn't allowed to fly in helicopters contracted to the military anyway—I worked for the Red Cross, and the Red Cross is always neutral.

After the storm, I put a hold on any further trips to the Weather Coast until we could sort out the security protocols. I employed my training as a surf lifesaver in Queensland and some basic common sense to figure out what we needed: an emergency positioning beacon on the boat, plus waterproof radios and satellite phones. I realised none of the team members had boat licences, so I got them proper training and documentation, and I spent the next couple of weeks getting the boat kitted out with proper Pelican cases, dry bags and lifejackets. The relaxed Islander vibe was great, in its way, but it was no good if somebody got killed.

There was a small tourist scene in Honiara, but it wasn't like Fiji or Vanuatu; people mostly passed through on their way out to other islands. There were a couple of nice restaurants in town, a few fairly average hotels and a decent-sized expat community.

A couple of the helicopter pilots were into scuba diving, like me, and we would often rent gear and go diving on the weekends. I had started scuba diving at the end of high school, but it became more of a habit when I was in the field. When I went on my rostered rest-and-relaxation trips, I was generally alone, and diving was something I could do by myself that helped to pass the time. Some of the most beautiful scuba diving spots in the world are in remote locations, but they are easily accessible when you're working remotely. I got my advanced diving licence in Egypt during a rostered break from Yirol, and did some of the best diving of my life in Port Sudan, on the edge of the Red Sea. In South Africa, I went diving in a beautiful kelp garden to watch seals frolic in the water. It was incredible, until I realised that I was in a Great White shark hunting ground, and I looked pretty seal-like in my 11-millimetre wetsuit.

The diving around the Solomon Islands was pretty spectacular. The Islands had seen a lot of action during the Second World War and there were quite a few military wrecks sunk off shore, including a massive Japanese submarine just near one of the beaches of Guadalcanal. The sub had come under attack by a New Zealand naval ship and both vessels, badly damaged, had been forced to beach themselves on the island. The sub had then slipped 10–15 metres under the water, hull almost intact except for where the nose had snapped off; you could dive right down through the middle of the boat, to a depth of 30 metres. Off Gizo, we dived the wreck of a Hellcat fighter plane which was rumoured to have been JFK's plane during the war. I'm not even sure he was a pilot, but the wreck was very cool.

When I wasn't diving, I spent my free time exploring hidden coves and private beaches, swimming in the emerald water in a place that felt like paradise. Again, I thought, *this humanitarian aid lifestyle is pretty sweet*, but the Solomons was the end of that dream for me. I'm glad I made the most of my few months on the Islands, because it was the last time I worked somewhere so relaxed.

In addition to the Weather Coast project, I also worked in Malaita, another island north-east of Guadalcanal. Over many, many years, the people of Malaita had stacked piles of coral on the seabed to create artificial islands just off the coast, building houses and schools in the middle of them, and a church, as a monument to God. Some of the artificial islands were over a hundred years old and they were linked by pathways of coral that were raised up out of the sea. It reminded me of *Waterworld*, the Kevin Costner movie. Quite a beautiful place to visit.

Unfortunately, the communities on the artificial islands had nowhere to grow food, and no safe harbour in a storm. There was tension with the communities that lived on the mainland, which made it difficult for the islanders to access any natural resources. The Red Cross had noticed a high mortality rate among the kids on the artificial islands, too, which was in part because they were so far away from the nearest health clinic. It wasn't a long boat journey back to shore, but if the men had taken all the boats out fishing, or it was dark, the wait could be deadly for a sick kid.

We were able to do very simple things to help these communities, like getting them to keep a store of coconuts on the island so they could give the milk to the children when they were dehydrated. We also worked on reconciliation programs between the islanders and the people on shore so that they'd have somewhere to go when storms were brewing, or when tsunamis were forecast. The far-northern Solomons had experienced a tsunami a few months before I'd arrived. I didn't think the artificial islands could withstand an earthquake, let alone a tsunami.

We would stay a night or two on the islands each time we visited to get a feel for the local community. They weren't easy places to live—a bit of rock in the middle of the ocean, with no modern comforts at all, but no one said hygiene promotion work was easy. The diet of two-minute noodles and Spam continued, but this time without the supplementary pineapple and coconuts.

To shower, I'd jump into the ocean; there was no other option. Going to the toilet was a whole different matter. Space on the island was at a premium and that did not include real estate for toilets. A series of wobbly planks, about a metre above the ocean, led to a small outcropping of coral about thirty metres out into the sea. At the end of the plank, there was usually (but not always) a small privacy screen, behind which there was a small platform. When it was time to go, you hung your bare arse over the platform and let your waste fly into the ocean.

If you'd been trained since the age of two to walk over the slippery planks and hang off the platform, it was pretty easy, but I hadn't. At high tide, there was at least water to fall into either side of the walkway, but at low tide there was exposed rock and coral, which was very likely covered in faecal matter. As a nurse, walking along the slippery planks while worrying about falling into shit-covered coral was daunting. It was to be avoided unless absolutely necessary. All bowel movements were timed with the tide.

One night when I was staying on the artificial island, I woke up at about 4 a.m. desperate to go to the toilet. I was a guest in someone's house, alone in one room, but on the other side of the door there were six people sleeping on the floor who I'd have to step over to get outside. I'd then have to make my way in the dark through a very small village where everyone lived on top of one another, across the island to the plank of death, then across to the platform on the other side. I lay awake for what seemed like hours trying to convince myself I didn't need to go to the toilet. Eventually, I decided to drink all the water in my water bottle and pee into that instead. I knew it would be weird if my host family heard me, but that was just the chance I had to take. I had to smuggle a litre of urine out of the house and dispose of it subtly the next morning.

I stayed in Malaita for a couple of weeks while the Red Cross team worked with the community there, and it was a little more comfortable than on the artificial islands. I worked out a deal with the local kids where I traded batteries for shellfish, which was a welcome break from Spam. For a couple of days, I was able to swap DD batteries for live lobster and crab, but then my seafood connection ran dry. The woman who was hosting me in Malaita felt quite bad about it, so she went out of her way to organise a crab feast for dinner one night. A 'crab feast' turned out to be just two crabs shared among the whole family, and as the guest of honour I was given the crab roe. I hated crab roe, but what could I do? It was so generous of them to give me the prized, squishy guts. I mixed it with two-minute noodles and forced it down, with a grateful smile on my face.

After a few weeks, I started to wonder if people could go mouldy. Between being wet from the rain, the humidity and showering in my clothes more often than not, the fungal infection that I had first picked up in Nepal had turned into a series of abscesses. I had had one abscess a week develop since I had arrived in the Solomons, so I'd started to shower myself in Dettol, trying to clear out whatever organisms had decided to take up residency on my chest and neck. During my last trip to Malaita, an abscess I had been nursing on my chest began to grow. I suspected it was pretty nasty, but it was hard to get a proper look because the house where I was staying had no electricity and the rooms were very dark. I got a head torch out and tried to examine it in the flaky old bathroom mirror. No dice. I then tried taking photos of it—my first disgusting selfie! The abscess was red with a green centre, and the redness looked to be spreading towards my shoulder. It felt soft but had a hard core, which was a bit alarming. I also had a low-grade fever. Things didn't look good.

I needed some treatment, but the local clinic was closed and I couldn't find the local Red Cross staff, so I decided to manage it myself. I just needed to open the thing up and give it a good clean, I thought. But for that I needed light. I needed to see what I was doing. I decided to go outside and detach the rear-view mirror from the Red Cross car and take a look at my gross abscess in the bright sunshine.

I balanced the rear-view mirror on the rear tyre of the car and pulled a razor blade out of my first-aid kit, then sliced right through the middle of the ulcer. It was partially successful. I managed to liberate some of the toxic pus, but the cut hurt so much that I felt dizzy. I was weak at the knees, so I decided to move the operation inside again. I'd have to dig around in there to get the green head out. If I was going to pass out, it should probably be indoors.

Inside, armed with the rear-view mirror, my head torch and pair of tweezers, I went at it again. Feeling sick and almost blind with pain, I managed to get hold of the green head of the abscess, which I had assumed would be a small ball like the head of a pimple. Actually, it was more like a root. When I finally pulled the bugger out, I had a hole in my chest the size of a cigarette butt and I was holding onto the bathroom sink to stop myself from keeling over.

What I had, as it turned out, was a tropical ulcer. They were quite common in the Solomons because of the sun and the damp, and they weren't life-threatening if they were treated. But I got eight of these ulcers over the next seven weeks and it became pretty annoying. I dealt with each of the little buggers in turn, until finally one appeared on my face. Not even I was stupid enough to try and perform surgery on my own face. It was time to admit defeat.

A couple of weeks shy of the end of my contract, I left the Solomon Islands and went home to get myself on a serious course of antibiotics. This was the first exotic disease I managed to pick up during my career. Unfortunately, it wouldn't be the last.

# 10

# WHAT WOULD RAY MARTIN SAY?

In November 2007, Cyclone Guba tore through south-east Papua New Guinea, killing at least 149 people. The torrential rains caused major landslides and flooding, washing away bridges, roads and dozens and dozens of houses. Another 200 people died in the aftermath of the storm, drowned in the floods, and thousands of people were displaced.

I went back to my studies after the Solomons, and looked for short missions until something more substantial came up. A friend who was now working with Oxfam gave me a call to ask if I was interested in helping out in Papua New Guinea, assisting with the water and sanitation component of Oxfam's emergency response. It was just a couple of weeks after the cyclone had hit and I'd never worked that kind of mission, so I was keen.

Another friend of mine, Emma, had done a lot of work in PNG. She was an HIV adviser with a lot of experience in the field and I respected her opinion. She had told me some horrific stories relating to local practices and HIV transmission: men slicing open their penises to insert pearls under the skin for sexual pleasure; a widespread culture of gang rape that was deemed socially acceptable. The work was obviously intense, but overall I got the impression that she enjoyed working in Papua New Guinea.

I texted Emma to let her know I was headed to that part of the world. *That's great*, she replied, *but where are you going? I hope it's not Popondetta*. Emma had worked all over the world, in Ethiopia and Eritrea, so I thought of her as a real humanitarian badass. I asked her why Popondetta was a problem, since that was in fact where I was going. *It's the only place I've ever been frightened*, she wrote. *I would never go back.*

Emma went on to explain that the palm oil industry was fuelling intense violence in that part of Papua New Guinea. The industry was worth millions and workers were paid well to plant and harvest, but that money went straight to the gambling dens and bars of Popondetta. On payday, that influx of money translated into drinking, anarchy and disorder.

My dad had worked in Papua New Guinea and he told me a different set of stories, about landing planes on the sides of mountains and trekking through the jungle. It was all mixed up with things I read about Anzacs on the Kokoda Trail, marching through the tropical heat with their rifles on their backs, driving the Japanese invasion back to the northern sea. My grandfather had been posted there during the Second World War, which made me really curious to see the place. Besides, I didn't think it could be any worse than Aurukun.

Popondetta is near the port of Oro Bay on the north coast of Papua New Guinea, directly across from Port Moresby if you head slightly north-east. It's the start of the Kokoda Trail, which runs nearly 100 kilometres across a spine of mountains that cuts right through the middle of the country. Cyclone Guba came off the Solomon Sea and landed right on Oro Bay, but the real damage came when the rain hit the mountains. Vast illegal logging operations had left thousands of tree trunks loose on higher ground. When the cyclone hit, the flood of water washed the massive logs down the river systems. The waterfall of trunks caused horrific damage as it tumbled towards the sea, smashing apart entire villages that had been built next to the river. Guba didn't receive much international press, but the damage was incredible.

The Oxfam emergency response team had been in PNG for just over a month when I arrived and they hadn't had an opportunity to do much assessment work. Popondetta itself was almost completely shut down. Road access from Oro Bay was cut off and the port was badly damaged. The Popondetta airport was open but the bridge was out, so you had to take a four-wheel drive across the river and up the muddy bank to reach the town. The supply lines were cut off, so the supermarket shelves were bare and an effective alcohol ban was in place.

This was a blessing, as far as I was concerned. With no alcohol to fuel conflict, Popondetta was a peaceful, beautiful place. The locals were friendly, even though they were struggling. They had limited food to eat but they worked with us on the recovery effort to get the town functioning again. Then two days before I was due to leave, the supermarket reopened and alcohol was reintroduced into the community, and I saw the Popondetta that my friend Emma had seen. For those two days, we locked ourselves inside our hotel, behind two-and-a-half-metre fences topped with barbed wire, and listened. People were partying, drinking and having fist fights—just like Aurukun on a Friday night. It sounded as though there was a riot going on outside.

But anyway, up until that moment, there were no issues. There was only the cyclone damage. The villagers who were affected weren't necessarily expecting help because this wasn't an area where the government or aid organisations flew in regularly to deal with crises, so people had already started rebuilding. They were surprised to see us, so when we offered to help or to give them supplies, they were also incredibly grateful.

With the roads washed out or impassable, we did most of our work via boat or helicopter. My first assessment job involved travelling by helicopter into the mountains, to the head of the Kokoda Trail. As we flew over the countryside, I saw the incredible destruction caused by the logging run-off; giant tree trunks were matted along the waterways like piles of matchsticks. In reality, some of these trunks were wider than I am tall, so there was no chance of moving them. We couldn't even consider rebuilding. It was simply a matter of relocating people and starting over on empty land. Thankfully there was plenty of space in PNG, so we wouldn't have all the political and logistical issues that I had faced in Banda Aceh.

I spent three or four days assessing the villages up in Kokoda, staying overnight in huts and houses as a guest of the local people while I looked at their water supply and sanitation in the aftermath of the disaster. I visited the Kokoda Trail Museum while I was up there, too. However hard the conditions were that we were operating in, it was nothing compared to the slog and misery that the Anzacs had faced. I found out later that my grandfather had gotten malaria when he was out there, like many other soldiers in PNG. He'd never really talked about the war.

When the work was done, our team put the call out for a helicopter to take us back to Popondetta and spent the better part of a day standing in the middle of a football field, waiting for a chopper that never came. The following day, my teammate Liam decided to set off by car to assess another village in the area while I stayed put and waited for my ride. Eventually, it turned up—a Papua New Guinean defence force helicopter, piloted by a guy chewing the biggest hunk of betel nut I had ever seen.

'Should you be chewing betel nut while flying a helicopter?' I asked. It wasn't the most powerful drug in the world, but it was still a drug. The pilot just shrugged and grinned at me.

I'd been waiting nearly two days for the flight, so decided to take my chances. I just said a prayer and strapped myself in. As we lifted off, the pilot asked if I had seen the fallen logs clogging up the river. 'You want to do a damage assessment? I'll show you some damage,' he said. He followed the line of the river all the way back to Popondetta, flying at a 45-degree angle to the earth and skimming over the landscape. The floor beneath my feet was Perspex and I was tipped forward along with the chopper, the tree-choked river rushing past under my toes. The pilot was a total cowboy—I actually thought I was going to die. I have to admit, though, I got some amazing photos.

We spent a lot of time in the northern part of the Oro Province, inspecting villages along the banks of the Kumusi River. The river looked like flowing chocolate because it was so polluted with run-off mud from the mountains. It had been the principal water supply for the communities along its banks, but it was useless now, too turbid to drink.

One of the communities I visited had moved to higher ground, to the top of a hill, but they had a limited water supply. We found a couple of springs in the area but the flow rates were very low; they'd have to hold a bucket under the spring all day to get enough water for the village. Instead, we worked on the idea of the sand filtration method of water collection where they could dig a hole close to the river so that the water would filter into it through the sand, removing enough of the impurities to make the water safe. Once I had taken them through the process, I told them I'd be back in a couple of days and we'd check how well the waterhole was working.

The village was built on a steep incline and the path up to it was slick with black mud, which made it a tricky climb. When I returned, the villagers came out to greet me with the traditional chant, 'Oro, oro, oro!' They met me at the water's edge and then danced backwards up the hill—it was considered impolite to turn their backs on me. They chanted as they went. They kept chanting as I trudged up the hill in my flip-flops, still chanting as I slipped and sliced my foot open on a sharp object buried in the mud. I looked down to see a huge gash covered in blood and black dirt, while the villagers continued, 'Oro, oro, oro!' It means 'welcome' in the local language.

At the top of the hill, I patched my foot up as best as I could and sat down with the villagers to talk water. The hole was full, they told me, but the water was not safe. 'What do you mean?' I asked. 'Are you feeling sick?' I couldn't think why the filtration wouldn't work, but the community insisted, the water was not safe.

With my bandaged and very sore foot, I managed to hobble back down the hill to visit the water point to see what was going on. I took a cup out of my pack, dipped it into the pool and had a drink. The pool that had formed wasn't covered so it wasn't totally sanitary, and I knew there was a fair chance with my delicate Aussie stomach that I'd end up with a bit of gastro, but I wanted to show the villagers it was okay. 'See?' I said, 'You can drink it.'

'Yes, but it's not safe,' they replied, staring out across the river. They pointed towards the other side and I followed their gesture.

There was a massive crocodile hanging out on the opposite bank. It was an absolute monster.

'He wasn't here before,' the villagers told me. 'But he has not moved since the cyclone. We can't send the children down for water, it is not safe.'

*Ahhhh*, I thought, standing there with my cup of water like an idiot, *it isn't safe*.

The villagers had to make do with the supply from the springs while I went back to Popondetta to work on the problem. (I also had to take care of my foot, which was looking a little gross.) At the cluster meeting the following afternoon, where the aid organisations working in the area met with the government and the police to talk about their various programs, I let everyone know about a giant crocodile that had interfered with my water campaign.

The local police were very happy to take care of the problem. They asked for fuel money and per diems for their staff, who would take a boat up to the Kumusi River and kill the crocodile. 'That's a very generous offer,' I replied politely. I was new to Oxfam, but I wasn't sure I could authorise a payment for crocodile hunting—I had learned my lesson from the Aceh ghostbusting incident. But I had to do something. What was the moral compass for this situation? I decided that I should think about how it would play out if it ended up on *60 Minutes*: what would Ray Martin say? In the end, I decided Ray would be cool with killing a crocodile if it meant people had access to clean water.

I told the police I couldn't write them a cheque for crocodile hunting specifically, but if they wanted to do a security patrol along the Kumusi River and they happened to find a security threat that they needed to deal with, Oxfam could contribute to that.

The next day, the police returned from their patrol to report that they had found a large crocodile and they had shot at it, but the bullets had bounced off its skull. They told me they needed a bigger gun. There were representatives from the PNG army in the meeting and they just laughed. They had the big guns; they could take care of it. Of course, the army would also require fuel and payment, so I wrote out yet another cheque for yet another security patrol. Thankfully, their weapons were up to the job.

We got a beautiful welcome at another village along the Kumusi River, where the villagers constructed an entrance gate for us out of bamboo poles and palm fronds. They greeting us in traditional dress, with ornate headbands and necklaces carved out of boar tusks, and beautiful printed skirts. Some of them wore huge garlands of hibiscus flowers around their necks. And again, they chanted 'Oro, oro, oro!'

We had brought what the villagers in PNG referred to as 'cargo', which was any materials they couldn't find on the land, essentially. It wasn't anything special, just jerry cans and building supplies, but they were very grateful for what they saw as a generous gift. The villagers had built a small hut in anticipation of our arrival, so that we would have somewhere to sleep overnight. It was a slightly elevated structure made of bamboo and grass string and it looked like it had been built in about two hours. 'I can't sleep in that,' I told my team. 'It's not strong enough. I'll just sleep on the ground.'

'That would be very disrespectful, they built this specifically for you.'

'It's not strong enough!' I insisted, but I didn't want to be rude. The villagers continued chanting while I waved and smiled like the Queen, and they escorted me all the way to the door of the hut. I was having flashbacks to Nepal. I knew where this was headed.

I placed a foot on the lowest step leading into the house and felt the green bamboo bend underneath it. The second I lifted my other foot off the ground, the step snapped under my weight and my leg plunged through the hole.

'Fuck!'

The chanting stopped quite abruptly as the whole village gasped.

My leg was lacerated by bamboo and I could feel the blood starting to trickle down my calf but I gave them all a big smile. 'It's okay! I'm okay! It's fine!'

Two men abruptly left the scene, disappearing into the village. 'Where have they gone?' I asked, my leg still in the hole.

'They've gone to kill a pig.'

'They what?'

'They have embarrassed the village; they must kill a pig to apologise to you.'

'No! Tell them not to kill the pig! Don't kill the pig!' I said hurriedly. There weren't a lot of pigs left after the cyclone and they were valuable assets. It was like offering to burn down your house because you'd dinged someone else's car.

Once I'd gotten free of the bamboo step, I managed to catch up with the two guys and talk them out of the planned animal sacrifice, but they weren't happy about it. We settled on a compromise: they would throw me a party before we left. Instead of the pig, the villagers brought handicrafts for me, gifts to say 'thank you' and 'we're sorry about your leg', including an armband made of that indestructible blue packing tape. The women in the village wore similar bands around their biceps, but mine was a little snug; it wasn't going to go any higher than my forearm. A little old lady from the village tried her hardest to ram it up past my elbow, grinning up at me with her orange betel-stained teeth—*Come on, you great elephant*—but eventually she had to admit defeat. She pushed my arm into the air Rocky Balboa-style—*Yay, it's a bracelet!*—as if that's what she'd intended all along.

There was a very small humanitarian response to Cyclone Guba, though it was a big disaster for the area. The Oxfam program was pretty modest, and it rolled out relatively slowly, but the communities in the Oro Province got on with things in the meantime. I joked later that I would head to Oro when the next global health pandemic broke out. There was enough fish, fruit and vegetables and meat in the communities to sustain the population, and there were plenty of materials for shelter and the weather was warm. This was the type of place that doomsday enthusiasts dream about—self-sufficient to a fault. As long as you could survive the malaria and the crocodiles, it was a fairly decent quality of life.

During my six-week mission in Papua New Guinea, I helped to design better rainwater catchment systems and to clean up many of the local health clinics. We flew new water tanks into various communities via helicopter and installed them at the clinics to secure the water supply, protecting against the impact of future disasters. It was a very action-driven mission, as opposed to one where there are days and days of planning and strategy meetings before you get to work. And as always, action suited me just fine. I finished up feeling satisfied that I had made a decent contribution. There were no major incidents. I'd even managed to save the pig. And I almost avoided getting another tropical disease.

A couple of days before I was due to fly out, I developed a sore on the arch of my foot. It was an ulcer the size of a ten-cent piece, not red, but incredibly painful. I transited through Port Moresby on the way home, and another couple of days later I flew into Brisbane. By that stage, I couldn't keep my shoe on and I was having difficulty walking. I'd never felt anything like this intense, throbbing pain. I didn't know what it was, but I knew it was something. My colleague Liam had had a very similar lesion. When he had complained about how painful it was, I'd told him to man up. And then he ended up in hospital.

I arrived in Brisbane on Sunday and took myself straight into the local emergency department. I felt very silly, because I knew the wound didn't look very impressive, but I was really struggling to manage the pain. The nurse on duty looked at me much the same way I had looked at my colleague and said, 'There's a GP clinic down the road.'

'I know, but I need someone with experience in tropical medicine,' I replied.

'You need to get a GP to look at it first,' she said.

'Look, I wouldn't normally say this but I'm a nurse and I've got a master's degree in tropical medicine. I think I need to see one of the infectious diseases doctors.'

'Oh, you think so, do you?' she puffed, all but rolling her eyes.

I managed to convince her to get a doctor, who happened to be a guy who'd worked in Papua New Guinea. He took one look at my foot and asked me where in the country I had been based. 'I was in Oro,' I told him.

'Were you in the Kumusi River?'

'Yeah, I was.' That was where I'd sliced my foot open.

'I'd say you've got a Kumusi ulcer!' The doctor was very excited. He had worked at a clinic on the Kumusi and he had a lot of great memories, and he was really keen to talk shop. How was the recovery effort going? Was so-and-so still around? I steered him gently back to the subject of my excruciating pain.

The thing on my foot was a Buruli ulcer. It's caused by the same bacterium that causes tuberculosis and leprosy, and it can get very serious very quickly. The doctor wrote me a script for antibiotics and another one for Probenecid, which increases the antibiotic effect. They were like horse pills. I would be on the drugs for at least a month—he advised me to stay home while they took effect.

After a couple of days, I felt fine. I was scheduled to go back to Nepal on a follow-up mission with Concern Worldwide, and I decided that since I felt fine, I probably *was* fine, so I might as well go. I took my horse pills with me and worked for the better part of the month in Kathmandu with no issues at all. The lesion disappeared completely.

Just before I was due to return to Australia, I woke up in the middle of the night with a familiar excruciating ache. I had finished the course of antibiotics literally a day earlier, and the ulcer had grown back while I was sleeping. By morning, it was the size of a five-cent piece. The following day, it was as big as it had been when I first left Papua New Guinea.

The general rule when you're in the field is that you don't buy pharmaceutical drugs from local pharmacies because you don't know what's gone into them or whether they are counterfeit. But in this particular instance, I decided to roll the dice with the drugs available in Nepal. I couldn't face the doctor in Brisbane after ignoring his advice. Anyway, the Nepalese drugs worked fine. It took about three months to get rid of the ulcer, but eventually they worked just fine.

# 11

# THE DONKEY EXPRESS

I wanted to work in disaster response. I was very clear about that. But I had applied a couple of times for the Red Cross's Field Assessment Coordination Team (FACT) training, which was the gateway to joining their emergency response roster, and I hadn't been selected yet. They only took a couple of people a year. If I waited around for an opportunity to come up with Red Cross, I could be waiting a while. Meanwhile, Concern Worldwide was looking for an emergency program coordinator and I was asked to apply for the job.

Concern is Ireland's largest humanitarian aid organisation, founded in 1968. It is involved in long-term development work, but also disaster and emergency response, and it has a team of permanent staff on call around the world. In the event of a disaster, the emergency response team is deployed within forty-eight hours, generally to support the Concern offices that are already embedded and operating in-country. The emergency missions are short, relative to some humanitarian projects, but they are high impact. The scenery is always changing. This is where I wanted to be.

The core emergency response team at Concern was very well established by the time I arrived, a multi-disciplinary unit that could be deployed quickly to run a full-scale operation in the event of a major disaster. They had a finance person, senior operations managers, water and sanitation experts and a human resources manager, but they wanted to add someone with public health expertise to the unit. I didn't have the exact qualifications the Concern team were looking for—I only had three years' experience in the field and they wanted five. I didn't have experience running budgets and logistics for a whole-of-country program—but they saw something in my CV that interested them. Though the emergency response was very different, I think it helped that I had worked for them as a consultant in Nepal, and I did well in the first two rounds of interviews. I flew all the way to Dublin for the final interview but it only lasted eight minutes.

'We just wanted to check that you don't have two heads,' they told me.

After I was hired, I would return to Dublin for semi-annual team meetings where I got to know this group quite well. They were a fascinating bunch—highly experienced, battle-hardened humanitarian aid workers who had been in the field for decades. Almost every one of them liked to drink, except for the director of the unit, Richard. Richard was a hulking giant who only ever drank English Breakfast tea, while the rest of them would happily visit five bars in a row on the hunt for the perfect pint of Guinness.

Eric was one of my favourites, a Swede in his early sixties who was an Energizer Bunny in the field but always fell asleep in meetings. He had left a thriving career as an engineer several decades earlier to move into humanitarian work and had been stationed everywhere over the years, including Iraq during the Gulf War. Eric was incredibly gruff. He didn't suffer fools easily, so I had to work hard and fast to earn his respect, but once I'd won him over, he treated me to endless tales of mischief and misadventure in the field. He was typical of many people in his line of work; he didn't wear his heart on his sleeve. The only thing that seemed to move him was poor engineering work. He'd get very angry about it, especially if it was ours.

Also on the team was David, an Irishman with an accent as thick as mud, who told stories about sitting on top of a truck driving down the streets of Mogadishu during the Black Hawk Down UN conflict, or sitting at his desk when a bullet came through the wall and hit a colleague standing next to him. Another guy, Roger, lived on a farm and made cheese in his spare time. He talked about dressing up in disguise to cross the border into Afghanistan without a visa during the Soviet–Afghan War.

These were people who had been in humanitarian work before it was professionalised, before security became a primary concern. I wanted to impress all of them, but it was tough. They'd been everywhere, seen it all, in much tougher conditions than I would ever face. I joked with them that I could never catch up, because there were too many rules now, and they were the ones who were policing them. David and Roger were largely office-based by the time I met them. Roger was in charge of disaster risk reduction programming, which was long-term strategic planning rather than coalface emergency work. They would both deploy very short term for major disaster scenarios, but as with the rest of the most senior team members, they were focused on the big picture in a global sense.

The country director on the emergency response team was a woman named Emily, and like me she had started out as a nurse. She had decades of experience under her belt, too. She had deployed and acted as country director for Concern in many disaster and relief scenarios, and she was incredibly open and generous with me when it came to sharing her experience. Sophie, who was the emergency finance manager on the team, brought a different kind of expertise. She came from a banking background, but had taken a five-year sabbatical from her career to devote herself to humanitarian work. She was a very maternal figure—loved having the whole team over for dinner—and she was a gun when it came to figuring out how to move aid money around in unstable countries that had no banking systems or ATMs.

What I appreciated most about the Concern team was that they were always looking for ways to do the job better. I think it was a very Irish sensibility, super self-critical. For me, it was an incredible learning environment that pushed me to excel. Could we have hit another 50,000 people? Could we have delivered these programs in a more integrated way? What else could we have done? It was very different to what I had experienced in the Red Cross, where more weight and attention was focused on achievements than failures.

Concern was also doing what I considered to be the shittiest but most rewarding work. The organisation had a mandate to focus on the twenty poorest countries in the world, and the poorest districts of those countries. In the four years I would work for them, I was sent to the crap holes of crap holes, truly terrible environments, but I knew that my work was having an impact where it counted most. And I really tried to make it count.

After I got the job, I was on call almost year-round. Whatever plans I might have made got swept aside when disaster struck. I got the call and was on a plane within forty-eight hours. The missions were supposed to be a maximum of three months, but they never worked out that way—it was always longer. And when I wasn't living in tough, demanding conditions, I was constantly in transit, sitting in shitty airport lounges. Under the circumstances, it was virtually impossible to maintain a normal life. Relationships were especially difficult. I burned through three partners while I was working for Concern, including one who dumped me via a satellite phone six weeks into my first mission. The call was costing me three dollars a minute, and I was literally holding starving black babies in my arms when it happened. I got no points for being a humanitarian hero.

My first placement for Concern was in Ethiopia, west Africa. Concern had a local team working on long-term malnutrition and agriculture development programs but there was a food security crisis on the horizon and I was sent as additional support to head it off before it got out of control.

Food security was a seasonal issue in Ethiopia. The Hunger Season came around every year when food supplies from the previous harvest ran out, but the situation we were looking at in 2008 was outside the normal cycle. There had been a drought, and malnutrition rates were rising. In countries where food security is an issue, humanitarian agencies keep track of the Global Acute Malnutrition (GAM) rate, and anything over 10 per cent of the population is considered a crisis. This is where things were headed in Ethiopia, so Concern was expanding its program. My job was to support the local team to reach new parts of the country.

There are two types of malnutrition. One is called 'stunting', which means you're too short and too small for your age. This is a result of long-term malnutrition—the kind of issues I saw in Alice and Aurukun. The other form of malnutrition is 'wasting', which is an acute problem caused by not having enough food *right now*. A child with wasting malnutrition can be quite tall, developmentally normal, but they are just too skinny—skin and bones. Stunting malnutrition will disadvantage a child in that it will affect their brain function and physical performance over time, but wasting malnutrition will kill them.

Once upon a time, kids suffering wasting malnutrition were treated in hospital, fed through a tube over three or four weeks until they were out of danger. It presented a huge opportunity cost for the mothers, as they were away from their older, more robust children and their fields weren't being planted or harvested. Many mothers would leave with their child as soon as they improved just a little, for completely understandable reasons, but it would endanger the malnourished kid in the long term. Screening of malnourished children was also problematic, historically, because it involved taking cumbersome gear from village to village to weigh and measure every child. It was a slow process, which meant that kids weren't being referred to the clinic until their malnutrition was fairly advanced.

By the time I arrived in Ethiopia, the protocols had changed dramatically, beginning with the way that kids were assessed. Médecins Sans Frontières (MSF) had figured out that no matter how big or small a child was, the fat on their arms was roughly the same thickness. When a child lost weight, they lost fat from the backs of their arms, so measuring the circumference of their arms was a very good way to determine if they were malnourished. MSF developed a special tape to measure a child's mid-upper arm circumference: MUAC tape. It was colour-coded red, yellow and green, which helped volunteers in the community to classify children quickly. Green was okay, yellow meant moderate acute malnutrition and red indicated severe acute malnutrition. Kids who measured yellow or red were referred into the Concern program.

The way that children with malnutrition were treated had also changed over time. In the mid-1990s, a development and nutrition specialist by the name of André Briend was watching his kids eat from a jar of Nutella when he had a flash of inspiration. He developed a product called Plumpy'Nut, similar to peanut butter, that was resistant to bacteria, very high in calories and didn't need refrigeration. Plumpy'Nut could be distributed easily and administered by parents in the home. You didn't need clean water, you didn't even need clean hands; kids could just tear off the corner of the packet and suck the Plumpy'Nut right out. In the Concern program, kids who were diagnosed with moderate malnutrition were treated with corn soy blend (CSB), a vitamin-enriched flour that was mixed with oil to make a high-calorie porridge, and kids with severe malnutrition got the Plumpy'Nut.

When severely malnourished kids were referred to us, we'd start their treatment with something called the Appetite Test. Their immune systems were often so repressed that we couldn't tell if they had any other serious medical conditions that needed attention, so we would give each kid a packet of Plumpy'Nut to see if they were interested in eating. (Nothing has ever made me quite as happy as the sight of sixty starving kids each sucking on a packet of very sweet peanut butter with huge grins on their faces.) If the test went well, we sent the mothers home with two weeks' worth of Plumpy'Nut, and we kept tracking their progress and administering the food until the kid was back in the safe zone.

Kids who didn't pass the Appetite Test were admitted to hospital, for roughly four days. The kids often had malaria or pneumonia, sometimes tuberculosis or HIV. The more time we kept the kids in, the more chance there was of cross-contamination. Our job was to get the kids to gain weight, or to refer them on for more extensive healthcare. In our hospital, we fed them a milk-based product called F75 and sometimes they got antibiotics or blood transfusions, but the medical care was by necessity very basic: their systems were incredibly fragile. The blood volume in these very weak kids was so low that an IV drip could send them into cardiac arrest. I learned this the hard way at the beginning of my mission—malnutrition kills in many different ways. We lost more kids in the first ten days I was in Ethiopia than I had in my entire nursing career.

I was based in Shashogo in south-west Ethiopia, in the Southern Nations, Nationalities, and Peoples' Region (SNNPR). It was several hours' drive from Addis Ababa, on the ridge of the Rift Valley, close to where the oldest human skeleton had been discovered.

We decided to set up operations in Shashogo because of the number of malnutrition cases that were presenting in the area. The town had a small hospital where we could operate, plus a larger hospital an hour and a half away where we could refer critically ill patients, and there was a network of clinics in the local area that could refer malnutrition cases to us.

I was assured that the hospital in Shashogo was well-equipped and running properly, but there were a lot of things that troubled me about its operations. Critically ill kids were crammed in one room, sharing mattresses on the floor, and the general level of cleanliness was troubling. The local nurses didn't seem to be following protocol for patient care, either, and almost every day when I arrived another kid had died. The attitude to this was less urgent than I would have liked. *What's the big deal? Children die in this country.*

On the fourth day after I had arrived, an infant presented with something called nystagmus, which means that their eyes moved rapidly from side to side, involuntarily. I had never seen it before. In this case it could have been a symptom of several different things; it could have been a convulsion or a brain injury, or something as simple as an electrolyte imbalance. Maybe it was a symptom of sodium deficiency? I wasn't sure, we had no access to a lab to do a test. I didn't have the means to research it. There was no internet in Shashogo and the phone reception was terrible. The local nurses told me the condition meant that the baby was about to die. They said that it had happened before in the clinic and there was nothing more they could do. I figured I might as well try something rather than nothing at all. I mixed a little salt and water and spoonfed it to the infant. Sadly, within five minutes, the baby had passed away. I didn't know if it was because of my treatment, or if it would have happened anyway, but I was upset that it had happened at all. I was frustrated by my lack of knowledge, so I made a decision to make sure I had proper resources in the field in future. I started creating a library of downloaded reference material that I could take with me wherever I went. I couldn't be an expert on everything, but I could be well armed.

In addition to wrapping my head around the clinical program, I had a lot of meetings with local stakeholders as I worked to put a plan together for the program expansion around Shashogo. I had to meet with local police, the mayor, local clinics and hospital managers, as well as representatives from Ethiopia's food and agriculture and health departments.

It was very tough going, for reasons that I didn't anticipate, because I had never worked in such a fraught political context. The Ethiopian government was corrupt and controlling, prone to harassing civilians and political opponents, and determined to suppress the truth about health and environmental problems in the country. When there was a cholera epidemic in Ethiopia aid organisations were forced to call it 'acute watery diarrhoea' and we weren't allowed to use the word 'malnutrition' when talking with government representatives. We weren't permitted to speak openly about the number of malnutrition cases we were seeing, because the government was extremely invested in controlling people's perceptions. A government that could not feed its people was obviously not a good government, and the legacy of Bob Geldof and Live Aid meant that Ethiopia was still a punchline for jokes about starving children. Malnutrition wasn't good for business, so as far as the Ethiopian government was concerned there *was* no malnutrition crisis.

Working with the government involved a diplomacy that really drove me nuts. I preferred being direct and honest about the situation and I saw a lot of harm in what they were doing, directed at their own people. I didn't quite know the best way to manage the situation. Between this, and the high infant mortality rate at the hospital, I started to feel quite anxious. I wasn't sleeping very well and I began to have shortness of breath and a dry mouth, which morphed into a sense of unease and panic. I really didn't feel right, and I started to think that maybe I wasn't cut out for the work. Maybe my other overseas missions had just been a fluke? I didn't understand it. I had been very relaxed in the past.

It took me a good couple of weeks to realise that the problem was the coffee. I was smashing four macchiatos a day. Coffee was part of the culture in Ethiopia. Every meeting started with coffee and it was rude not to accept it. The problem was, I was the only nurse I knew who didn't mainline the stuff—I usually didn't drink it at all. Four espressos a day were sending me over the edge—tachycardia, dry mouth, insomnia. I wasn't having panic attacks, I was overdosing on pure, high-grade caffeine. The minute I started sneaking cups across to my interpreters, the feelings of panic went away. The politics were still a pain in the arse, of course, but politics were the least of my problems. As long as I had sick kids to worry about, they weren't going to get in the way. I found ways to talk about the crisis without referring to it directly, and writing reports in a subtle way that enabled me to do what I needed to do. We talked about food security instead of malnutrition, community support instead of crisis, and the government officials nodded their heads and let us get on with our work.

The drought didn't look like a drought. The issue wasn't that there hadn't been any rain, but that the rain hadn't come at the right time, so the landscape wasn't one of cracked and scorched earth. In fact, by the time we started rolling the program out around Shashogo, we were battling with wet weather and floods. For the communities, the rain threatened the remaining food supply because it could destroy the new crops. For us, it meant that travel was very difficult.

We had a distribution plan that involved moving stores of Plumpy'Nut out to some of the remote clinics, but access was nearly impossible over muddy flood plains and valleys. The best bet was to travel by donkey, but it was slim pickings in the donkey market; the animals were as badly affected by malnutrition as the people were. I wasn't convinced they could carry a loaf of bread, let alone a box full of Plumpy'Nut, but the owners insisted they were up to the job. We would be providing their animals with extra food, of course. Donkey malnutrition treatment became our little side project.

About half of the locations we had to visit were on the floor of the Rift Valley. When we set off into the field, we rode in carts attached to the back of the donkeys with boxes of Plumpy'Nut stored in the trunk behind us. I felt terrible about it because I was so much bigger than the average Ethiopian and I was convinced I was going to give the donkey a heart attack. Whenever the terrain got a little tricky and the beast slowed down, I jumped out of the carriage and walked. I ended up walking or jogging alongside the donkey almost as much I was in the cart.

On one of these trips, we came to a wadi, a kind of natural river dam with patches of dry land cutting through big pools of water. The road went straight through the middle of the wadi, but my colleague, Sister H—, and I decided to hop out and walk around the edge of it, to meet the donkey on the other side. The road across the wadi was a little precarious. It would be an easier journey without us in the cart, we figured. On the way back from the delivery, the driver insisted that we should both stay in the cart to cross the wadi, that everything would be fine, but I politely declined. Sister H— didn't want to get her feet muddy again, so she elected to stay with the driver. Not a good choice, as it turned out.

When I was halfway around the wadi, a good hundred metres away, I saw the cart flip at a precarious angle and slide backwards into a giant pool of muddy water. The poor donkey, hitched to the cart, was dragged along with it. I broke into a sprint to reach the accident but the animal was sunk up to its chest by the time I got there, and the driver was hollering desperately in a language I didn't understand. I jumped straight into the water to grab hold of the donkey and felt mud rising up to my knees, thick, heavy and sticky. The water was up to my mid-thigh and the donkey's head was resting on my shoulder. He was thrashing around, but obviously quite stuck, and all I could do was try to soothe him while the driver struggled to de-rig the cart.

Sister H— had scrambled for dry land as soon as the donkey

had hit the water, but some women from neighbouring houses had heard the commotion and they had come running to our aid. It took four of us to get the animal unstuck and back on the road, at which point it trotted happily away. I was still stuck, unfortunately. The women had to pull me out of the water next. At least three of them were tugging on my arms until the mud finally slurped away. They were so fantastic. They disappeared for a moment then came back with tin cans full of water and started washing the mud off my boots and legs, fussing despite my protests that I was fine.

As I was standing there thinking about how surreal all of this was, I got stung on the eyelid by a bee.

The list of unusual problems continued. The locals started to view Plumpy'Nut in the way Australians view Red Bull, as a quick burst of energy that could get them through the day. It was especially popular with guys working as manual labour for a minimum wage. The demand created a black market for Plumpy'Nut, which created temptation for the mothers in our program. The mothers would sell a small amount of their allocation to traders and traders would on-sell it at the market at an inflated price.

It was easy to game the system. We kept a graph of the height and weight of children involved in the program, with a line that clearly demarcated a healthy weight goal. Once kids crossed that line, they were given a two-week supply of Plumpy'Nut and discharged from the program. Unfortunately, because the program had been running for so long in Ethiopia, the mothers knew how to sail under the radar. They would feed their child the Plumpy'Nut until they came close to the line, then reduce the supply to reduce the kid's weight again, selling the extra supply to raise money for their families. As a result, we often saw wave patterns on the weight charts, bobbing up and down under the discharge line.

The problem was in part cultural. Our program was for children under the age of five, but those kids lived in households where everyone was starving. Families in Ethiopia ate off the same large plate, so the idea of feeding the child but not the other children or the adults was a big leap, conceptually. The mothers were simply doing their best to provide for the whole family, but it put an extra burden on the malnutrition program that in turn put the whole program at risk. It was also no good for the kids. They weren't recovering without their full rations, with their lifesaving weight gain plateauing and sometimes even reversing. We worked with the local government to try to manage the issue and they ended up passing a local by-law that made it illegal to sell Plumpy'Nut in the local markets. The food safety team responsible for checking the meat hygiene was now tasked with policing the Plumpy'Nut trade as well.

We had a similar issue with the corn soya blend given to the moderately malnourished kids: the oil that was used to mix their porridge started appearing on the black market as well. But rather than try to control the problem by policing it, we decided to pre-mix the CSB flour and oil and distribute it as a 'wet mix'. This had huge consequences for our program. Instead of handing out flour and oil once a month, it meant mixing the oil and flour on site before we handed it out, after which it would only keep for two weeks. In addition to hand-mixing tonnes of CSB every month, we had double the number of distribution runs. It became a massive operation for the Concern team in Shashogo and I spent a lot of my time on the mission up to my elbows in flour.

We had decentralised distribution points all around the region, based out of government warehouses, and the days when we went out to distribute the food were some of my best in Ethiopia.

The women would arrive in beautiful printed skirts, and gather to talk, or sometimes sing, while we weighed and measured the kids. The weighing was done in a makeshift tripod with a plastic laundry bucket suspended underneath, with the little kids laid naked inside the bucket.

As long as the line moved quickly, the atmosphere was lovely, though hot weather and hungry families could sometimes make the situation tense. The women were walking for two or three hours to get to the distribution site. When they had their CSB allocation, it was another two or three hours' walk home. Once, a family was attacked by a hyena, which killed one of the children. There were serious risks and challenges involved in getting something for free.

Difficult politics, malnourished donkeys, killer bees, black markets and packs of hyenas meant constant challenges, but the biggest challenge remained the rain.

We got a call from one of our remote clinics to say that they were on the verge of running out of Plumpy'Nut, even though they had a distribution scheduled for the following day. There would be major issues if mothers walked all the way to the clinic only to find that there was nothing waiting for them.

The clinic was a two-and-a-half-hour drive from Shashogo and all I had for the trip was a dual-cab ute. It wasn't quite as robust a vehicle as I would have liked for that environment, but it would have to do.

I set out with a driver and a member of the local team. We were fine on the way out, though it was late in the afternoon when we arrived. By the time we'd unloaded the ute and checked the supply charts at the clinic, it was coming up to five o'clock. We had an hour and a half of sunlight left for a two-and-a-half-hour drive home. On top of that, one of the local nurses came and told us we should stay overnight because it was raining further up the valley. The sky was clear over our heads but there were very black clouds on the horizon, and she was worried that the water would flow down to the wadi we had to cross on the way home. But our driver assured us we had plenty of time.

We weren't more than a couple of kilometres out of town when we saw the head of the river forming in the distance. It looked very cool, the water beginning to roll over a dry landscape, at first just millimetres thick. But very quickly, the flow spread out across the entire plain, getting deeper and deeper as we tried to plough through it. It wasn't like a river with visible banks; it was water as far as you could see, ankle deep, and after a few minutes we were bogged in it.

We pushed and wriggled the ute along a bit further, then got stuck again. And again. Meanwhile, the water was rising towards our knees and the light had faded. It's not that we were anchored in the mud, necessarily, but we could no longer see the road. We decided to stop and wait for the water to pass; the driver assured me it would happen quickly. An hour later, the water had risen up above knee level.

The driver did some scouting and suggested we move the ute to the little rise of a hill close by, then wait out the flood overnight. We had no food and no communications. I had broken all of my own security rules because we had left in a hurry, but at least we were safe and dry. Then I realised I had to go to the toilet. I held on for what seemed hours, but in reality it was probably twenty minutes. I scanned the dark horizon. The rain was over our heads now and the water was flowing fast around the sides of the ute. Toilet options were limited. I climbed out of the window and balanced myself on the bumper, gripped the tailgate, hung my bare white arse as far out as I could and peed.

I then climbed back in the window, along with the last shreds of my dignity. This was a truly crap situation, I decided. We might be safe, but I was hungry and tired, and had no interest in climbing out the window the next time I needed to go to the toilet. I discussed our options with the driver and we settled on a different plan. We would walk back into the town we had just left, try to find somewhere to stay and then come back in the morning to see if we could get the ute out.

We made our way back across the flood plain in the rain and the dark, the water swirling around our calves, with no torches and, worst of all, no phone signal. The team in Shashogo didn't know where we were.

We knocked on the first door we found and the guys managed to negotiate some food and shelter for us, and dry clothes. Being a white giant, there were no regular clothes in the house that would fit me, but the family kindly supplied a yellow muumuu in wax print fabric, with bright orange lace around the sleeves. My final shred of dignity was now gone, but I was beyond caring. They gave me a bed to sleep on and thankfully I did not break it.

At sunrise, we walked back out to the ute. It was stuck deep in the sludge in the middle of a muddy plain, some kilometres away from the nearest dry stretch of road. We weren't going anywhere in a hurry. We ended up enlisting about thirty men from the town and calling in a LandCruiser from Shashogo, and over the course of about six hours, with a lot of pushing and digging and towing, we finally got ourselves and our car free of the flood.

Shashogo is a beautiful part of the world, but the living conditions were less than desirable. This was a short-term emergency mission. We weren't staying longer than a few months, so investing in accommodation was not a priority. Before I arrived, the team had taken up residency in a disused police station on the edge of town. It had no bathrooms or running water, so they were taking bucket showers under a tap in the backyard, and had managed to dig a very shallow pit latrine and hoist a bit of tarp around it. The team had hired a cook, and had instigated a system of pooling funds each week to buy supplies, contributing just enough to make a fresh batch of *injuria* (a fermented pancake) every few days. We slept on bunk beds in what I assume had been the holding cells of the police station, and I shared with Sister H—, who snored loud enough to make the bed shake.

I didn't want to be the expat who turns up and demands more creature comforts, especially when the mission would only run for a few months. I'd taken pride in my ability to rough it in the past, so I was determined to stick it out. I lasted about a week. I was hungry all the time, I couldn't sleep, and washing my naked white body in the middle of a freezing field became my least favourite part of the day.

The last straw came when the pit latrine filled up and spilled over the wooden foot plates. Beyond disgusting. I started walking two kilometres to the local hospital to go to the bathroom during the day, and squatted out in the open field at night. I could rough it, but this was too much, so I emailed the main office in Addis Ababa and got the green light to build a toilet and shower, and to hire another room in the police station to escape Sister H—'s nightly nasal symphony.

It took a good three weeks to complete the work on our bathroom and I was stuck with the moonlit scrub until then. To avoid losing my mind completely, I turned Sunday afternoon into a beauty therapy day, paying local women to come and wash my hair, and taking the time to shave my legs when there was enough sunlight to actually see them. The work I was doing was hard-going and sweaty, but the routine really helped me through it.

Unfortunately, I became a local attraction; everybody wanted to watch the white woman clean herself. It was kind of cute at first, but the attention quickly wore thin. I felt like a circus freak, with little eyes and faces peering at me through fence palings. The kids knew three sentences in English—*What is your name? What is the time? How are you?*—and they asked these three questions over and over again until I thought my head would explode. It didn't matter what I answered, there was no follow-up sentence.

I was the only white person in Shashogo, that was the problem. I was such a bizarre novelty I might as well have been covered in polka dots. It had been very different in Yirol because there was a whole team of expats in town and there had been plenty of white faces there before ours, but many of the people I encountered in Shashogo had never seen a white person before, or at least very few. And however weird it made me feel, they didn't feel weird about staring.

One day, I decided to visit the local market: several rows of tarpaulin squares spread out on the ground, covered in products and produce. At some point, as I wandered around, I realised I had grown a tail. Two or three people were following directly behind me, and behind them I had a crowd of admirers spreading out in a V forma-tion. When I moved, the crowd moved, walking over and across the market stalls, upsetting the fruit and vegetables as well as the stall-holders. I had inadvertently caused a mini riot and the local police were not happy. They strong-armed me out of the market square and asked me not to come back without a local staff member as an escort.

Shashogo was safe, and I was grateful for that. Every afternoon, I would go for a run to the edge of town, but after a few weeks the local kids cottoned on to my routine and started to join me.

There is really nothing more embarrassing than heaving along puffing while a bunch of Ethiopian children literally run circles around you. I would be beetroot red and pouring sweat, aching for a little peace and quiet, while the kids zipped around in figure eights, running off, running back—*What is your name?! What is your name?!*—then running off again. They thought it was very funny but I wanted to kill them. I actually picked up a rock one day and threatened them with it, like they were pigeons. 'Just stop it!' I shouted, mad with frustration. Then I realised what I was doing. *You're a paediatric nurse and you are about to throw a rock at some children*, I thought. *You really need to get a hold of yourself.*

It felt like I was living in a zoo and I was the main exhibit.

There were structural and cultural issues in Ethiopia that made the work frustrating as well. With vaccinations and health programs like ours running in the country, the infant mortality rate had come down but family planning was still geared around the idea that some percentage of your children would die. Overall, family sizes increased, putting an even bigger burden on already over-taxed national and natural resources. There were more people to feed and smaller parcels of land for each family to cultivate, which meant less food to go around all the time, not just in a drought. The kids weren't dying now but they weren't thriving either. We were on this treadmill of keeping kids alive long enough to get sick again the next season.

The malnutrition program was a bandaid for something that needed much longer-term intervention and strategic thinking, and long-term development work didn't suit my nature. I liked to feel as if I was fixing a problem before I moved on to the next one, but I just couldn't do that in Ethiopia. Other people were working on it, it wasn't my job, but I didn't really feel as though I was making an impact. When the problems are structural, and they run very deep, there's not a lot you can achieve in sixteen weeks.

For all of these reasons, and others not worth mentioning, I didn't enjoy my time in Ethiopia. Different people respond differently to different parts of the world, and that was one mission that just didn't suit me. Challenges are to be expected in this line of work, but I was getting it from every side, and the grind of it really wore me down in the end. I was more than happy to leave.

From a professional point of view, Ethiopia was very useful. I added malnutrition knowledge to my catalogue of experience alongside water and sanitation, primary healthcare and refugee camp development—an unusual mix. The more feathers I had in my cap, the more useful I could be in the humanitarian world. I felt like I was starting to see the big picture.

# 12

# I THOUGHT ONLY PIRATES GOT SCURVY

The Karamojong people of north-east Uganda are nomadic cattle herders. Historically, they were a marginalised group within Uganda, purposely excluded from development efforts by the national government and viewed as lesser people, rural and backward, by the rest of the population. They were armed, supposedly because they had seized military weapons after the fall of Idi Amin, and like the Dinka tribe in South Sudan, they fought brutally to protect their herds.

The Ugandan government was running a voluntary disarmament program in Karamoja, but relieving the Karamojong of their weapons left them vulnerable to raids from other tribes. The military couldn't protect the herds if they were dispersed, so they were moved into massive cattle camps while disarmament rolled out. As a result, the women and children in the region were separated from their primary source of nutrition. The cows and their milk were in one place and the women and their children were in another. This situation was exacerbated by a recent drought.

Médecins Sans Frontières had set up a malnutrition treatment program in the area following the drought, but it was a short-term intervention and it was coming to an end. The MSF Ugandan team knew there was an ongoing problem but they didn't specialise in long-term malnutrition, so they partnered with Concern to help transition the work over to the Ugandan government. I was sent to Karamoja, to an area called Nakapiripirit, to help with the transition.

Concern had an office just outside Kampala, run by a formidable Irish woman named Helen who had been with the organisation for twenty years. Helen had started out as a nurse, just like me, but she was now overseeing a number of complex programs in Uganda from a very well-established country headquarters. She hadn't visited Karamoja, however. Very few humanitarian organisations serviced the region because it was too unstable, and before we established operations in the area, we had to determine if it was safe.

Helen and I visited the UNDSS, the security unit of the United Nations, where we were briefed on the history and problems in the region. They told us that representatives of the UN World Food Programme had been killed in recent years when Karamojong tribesmen had fired shots into a moving car. The briefing we received was that the men were particularly dangerous if they'd returned from an unsuccessful cattle raid, when they would attempt to salvage their manhood by killing something or someone on the way home. The problem wasn't that people were being targeted, but that the violence was random. The UN was active in the region, but the teams were small and they travelled in bulletproof cars.

The final recommendation of the UNDSS was that we were safe to operate up there, but our team should probably wear bulletproof vests and helmets whenever we were travelling around. 'Okay, great,' Helen replied. 'Thanks for the brief.'

As we left the office she turned to me and said, 'They can be a bit overly dramatic. We don't need any of that stuff, don't worry about it.'

Uganda had been one of my favourite places on the truck tour that I had taken after leaving Alice Springs. I remembered national parks and rainforests, and the hills around Kampala. I remembered it as a picture postcard advertisement for Africa. For the most part, it was exactly as I recalled, though maybe a little busier. Wrapping around the shores of Lake Victoria, Kampala was dense and bustling—the traffic was appalling—but when we cleared Kampala's congested hills, the landscape opened up beautifully. Most of Uganda was lush and green. But Karamoja was a desert. The minute we passed Mount Elgon on our way north, the colour leached out of the earth.

Helen and I drove up to Nakapiripit together, using her personal driver. The Ugandan people were so terrified of the Karamojong that we couldn't convince anyone else to take us. In town, we found a tiny hotel that was essentially a community hall, with a little kitchen and a few dusty tables outside to serve as a restaurant. They served chicken and chips with a little slice of tomato when they could find it, or a local doughy bread called *foofoo* with a sauce of tinned tomatoes and oil.

The owner of the hotel was quite entrepreneurial. He had built tiny cement *tukuls* in the yard and called it the Nakapiripit Resort, thinking that once security improved he'd have a viable business. He was very happy to have us as guests. The rooms were quite nice inside, relatively speaking, with a bed, a shower cavity and toilet, though there was no running water. The hotel provided buckets of water for washing and flushing your waste away.

We set up our offices in the main building and started the assessment, visiting the clinic behind the Nakapiripirit hospital where MSF was operating. I hadn't worked with MSF prior to this but I was worried about the handover. They were known for being extraordinary in an acute crisis, but their exit strategy and transition to longer-term programming could leave people high and dry; at least, that seemed to be the general consensus. But in fact, the MSF team in Karamoja was amazing. The head of office was very experienced and very considered, and she wanted a robust plan in place before she handed over the program.

We spent a lot of time figuring out how to turn MSF's resource-intensive program into a model that would be sustainable in the long term. They had an expat doctor, two expat nurses, a logistician and a head of office, and we needed to scale back to a program led by a local team with weekly technical support visits from someone in the Concern team. MSF was particularly good at helping us with the language we needed to use with the Ugandan government to ease the transition from one model to another. MSF indicated that its team was leaving and suggested someone else might come in to support the program, but in the meantime the ministry of health should continue the work it was doing. We wanted the government to take ownership of the program before Concern offered to provide support.

The ministry of health knew what we were doing; it was more about getting the community and the local nurses on board. If the nurses thought Concern was operating a program, they would expect more pay for the additional work, whereas we wanted them to see it as part of their normal duties. The situation with the community volunteers was similar. MSF had been paying community volunteers US$80 a month to screen for malnourished children but it wasn't sustainable in the long term. It also wasn't a full-time job; it was more about keeping an eye on vulnerable kids in your own community. MSF had introduced the payment system because it had set up the program quickly in response to a food security crisis, but we had to find a way to reset expectations. In the end we decided the best way to do it was to let the program collapse for four weeks.

I left Uganda after the handover was complete and moved on to a mission in the Democratic Republic of Congo, but the following year I was recalled to Karamoja to run the Concern malnutrition program. I had a three-person team including two young Ugandan nutritionists and a driver, with the local Concern workers tasked with delivering the bulk of the care. We took over three rooms at the Nakapiripirit Resort, running a power generator to keep the operation going.

Karamoja was quite cold when I returned in April 2009. It was heading towards winter, so the landscape was a little greener, but my bucket shower was unbearably frosty in the mornings. I got into the habit of showering at lunchtime when the watery sun was at its peak.

There were nine or ten clinics around the region that were connected to the malnutrition program, some of them up to two hours' drive away, including one out on the Kenyan border in the west. I spent a lot of time crisscrossing the region with my team, getting to know the people and the landscape. I loved it out there.

The Karamojong people were incredibly beautiful. Like the Dinka in South Sudan, they were very dark-skinned and very tall, with lean, strong bodies draped in colourful beads and cloth. The babies wore strings of beads around their waists so that the mothers could see if they were growing. The women wore second-hand clothes or fabric draped over their shoulders.

Men took multiple wives in the region and the families were housed in communal villages designed with security in mind. The houses were surrounded by a two-metre-high fence made of thorny bush, with one small door in the fence set low to the earth. Inside, there was a second fence with a second door that wasn't aligned with the first. To access the village, you had to follow the space between the two fences until you reached the next opening. If cattle raiders attacked the village, this system could slow them down considerably. Unfortunately, it slowed me down, too. I could barely fit through the doors in the fences and was nowhere near flexible enough to shimmy under the way the Karamojong people did. I had to get down on my knees and crawl.

A few weeks into my mission, I started developing a peculiar kind of fever, which hit me only once a week and always in the middle of the night. Every Wednesday, I got a fever that made my legs feel like they were breaking, but by Thursday morning everything felt fine again. Initially, I treated myself with anti-malarial medication and assumed that it was working, but by the third round I figured it was something else.

I called Helen to let her know what was happening and she immediately called me back to Kampala. The last thing I wanted to do was sit in the back of a truck for five hours, but I had to admit I wasn't doing well. Of course, by the time I got to Kampala the fever had lifted again. I went to describe my troubles to a local doctor and he started writing a script before I was even halfway through. 'I know what you have,' he said. 'But you're telling the story so beautifully, please continue.'

When he told me I had brucellosis, I said it was impossible. 'I don't drink milk!' *I don't blow bubbles up cow vaginas either,* I thought to myself, thinking back to the young women of the

South Sudanese cattle camps. But the doctor assured me that it was inevitable with the number of cows in Karamoja. Every Westerner who visited the district came down with it sooner or later.

A child presented at the Nakapiripirit hospital during my mission who was in a very bad way, especially for her age. She was four or five years old but extremely thin, semi-conscious and hypoglycaemic. I worked with the nurses to try to stabilise her, including putting in a nasogastric tube. We even ran an IV drip, despite the risk of cardiac shock, because it seemed too dangerous not to.

I put a care plan together for the little girl, but I couldn't stay with her because security was quite strict. It was only a fifteen-minute drive back to the hotel, but that drive went over a ridge that was used by cattle raiders to move their herds and I wasn't allowed to cross it after dark. Helen was back in Kampala but she was having me call in every day because I was the only expat in the field. I was out there by myself, so she had to keep tabs on me. Anyway, I had left very specific instructions for the nurses, so I assumed everything would be okay. I took the IV out before I left because it required very specific observations and I didn't want to overwhelm the hospital team.

When I arrived back at the hospital the next morning, I saw a familiar scene: mothers who were involved in the malnutrition program sitting beneath a tree outside, chatting and feeding their children. Inside the hospital, I found the little girl, completely covered with a blanket. I assumed that she had died overnight and they were waiting for the mother to collect her body.

I wandered through the hospital looking for the nurses but the halls were empty. I found them at last in the kitchen, making tea. They were very surprised to hear that the little girl was dead. I hadn't checked the little girl's body, I had just assumed the worst, so I raced back to the ward to see if I was wrong. One of the local nurses raced along beside me. The child was most definitely dead, however; in fact she was in full rigor mortis, which meant the nursing team hadn't checked on her at all overnight.

To make matters worse, as I checked the corpse, the nurse went to the window and yelled in language, 'Whose child is this?' It was like that horrible scene in *Jaws* when all the kids scramble out of the water into their parents' arms and there's one mother left who can't find her kid, and realises slowly that her child was eaten by a shark. It was horrific. All the mothers clutched their babies and looked at the one woman in their midst whose arms were empty. The whole compound was silent as she stood up and walked into the hospital.

The nurse yelled at the mother for not taking care of her child but I really wanted to yell at the nurses for being derelict in their duty of care. I went through the notes on the chart but there was nothing. They hadn't given the girl any milk since I had left the night before. I stormed off to find the matron to figure out what the hell had happened, and fell into a frustrating conversation about how understaffed the hospital was in the evening.

When I returned to the ward, the child's body was gone and the nurses told me the mother had taken her home for burial. *Okay.* I turned my attention to the hospital protocols to figure out how we could stop it happening in future.

A couple of hours later, I was driving south towards one of the remote clinics when I saw the mother emerge from the scrub by the side of the road. I asked the driver to pull over so we could figure out what was happening. The mother was crying; she said the child was too heavy. Because the body had rigor mortis, she couldn't strap her to her back properly and the walk home was another three hours. She had left her child underneath a tree.

'This is not okay,' I said.

I asked the mother to lead me back into the bush to where she had left her child and I picked up the body. Her corpse smelled terrible: a mixture of death and the sickly sweet milk we had fed her that was still clinging to her clothes. I carried the little girl wrapped in a blanket back to the car and we drove her and her mother to their village.

The family was so grateful that we had brought the body back. They were so happy that they could bury their daughter at home. I didn't know what to say. I had never felt so inadequate.

As the malnutrition program rolled out, we began to suspect that malnutrition was far more widespread in Karamoja than we had ascertained. Merely anecdotally, the reports we were getting suggested that we weren't on top of the problem, but an opportunity came up that helped us to expand our net. We got word that the ministry of health was launching a polio vaccination campaign that would be incredibly well-resourced. About 300 staff members would be deployed to hit every house in the region, administering a few drops of polio medication to every child they encountered. I managed to convince the government to add MUAC screening to the campaign, with every child who came up red or yellow referred to one of our clinics. We were able to screen 135,000 kids for malnutrition in just three days.

I travelled around the region while the campaign was underway, checking on the teams and troubleshooting problems as they came up, and in one particular village in the north I discovered a whole new problem. As I watched the screening team doing the assessments, I noticed that every kid in the village had sores in the corner of their mouth. Many of them had mouth ulcers, too. I didn't know exactly what it was, but the mouth ulcers made me think of scurvy, because one of its symptoms was bleeding gums. I wondered if I was looking at some kind of micronutrient deficiency.

Micronutrients are the vitamins and minerals that you need to keep your body functioning—vitamins A, B, B1, C, D, et cetera. If you don't have enough variety of food or you don't get access to vegetables, you can develop a micronutrient deficiency, the most familiar of which is scurvy. Rickets is another one, which leads to bow-shaped legs. If these conditions sound old-fashioned, it's because they are.

I took photos of the kids with the mouth sores and sent them to the Concern nutritionist in Dublin, asking if I had actually found scurvy. To be honest, I was a little excited about the idea, only because the condition was now so rare. Only seafaring pirates got scurvy! I wanted to research it myself, but my internet access was limited to a USB dongle that only worked when I drove to the top of a hill a fair distance from our offices. Eventually, the Dublin team came back to me to say that it was probably a riboflavin or vitamin B1 deficiency. I had an MSF clinical handbook with me, so I looked up the symptoms and found that they matched perfectly.

A widespread riboflavin deficiency was still pretty rare—the last recorded incident in the journals that we could find was in 1951—so we notified WHO and the Centers for Disease Control and Prevention (CDC) knowing they'd want to do a formal assessment. They arrived, but two weeks later they still hadn't reached a conclusion. The operatives in the field knew what they were looking at, but WHO and CDC were slow-moving beasts and the investigation had to move through a bunch of formal stages. Meanwhile, I had a group of malnourished kids on my hands whose mouth ulcers made it too painful to eat.

I was also coming to the end of my mission in Uganda and I didn't want to leave the issue untreated, so I asked Helen for some extra funds to run an emergency response program. I made up little screening cards featuring pictures of the sores with categories one, two and three, to help us with assessment, then distributed copies of the cards to all the clinics in the region. Through the clinics, we did a mass distribution of multivitamins to anyone who was affected and because the kids got better so quickly, word spread, and more mothers presented. In the end, we were able to distribute vitamins to about 100,000 people in the space of four or five days.

When the WHO and CDC people came back to investigate the outbreak further, they were annoyed to find that everyone had been treated, so they couldn't collect any more useful data. *Too bad, you were too slow,* I thought. Later, they published a paper on the outbreak which complained that the research had been thwarted. As a nurse, though, I felt very confident that treating people was the right thing to do.

# 13

# TEA WITH COLONEL INNOCENT

I wrote an assignment during my master's course about refugee movement following the Rwanda genocide of 1994. Millions of displaced people had fled Rwanda into the Democratic Republic of Congo (DRC) and settled in a city near the border called Goma, where a huge cholera outbreak had occurred. Goma is located at the base of an active volcano and much of the land is covered in hardened lava, so it was very difficult to build latrines. Instead, the waste poured into nearby Lake Kivu, and the water was very quickly contaminated. Roughly forty-six people in every 1000 died, which triggered a major turning point in the way humanitarian agencies managed refugee settlements. The Sphere Standards that I had used in Banda Aceh were developed in the aftermath of Goma.

The movement of people across borders and political complications with the changing Rwandan government triggered conflict between DRC and Rwanda, as well as neighbouring countries. In the late 1990s, and for most of the last decade, the region was subject to ongoing wars and conflict. I had always known that the DRC was a humanitarian hot spot, but I didn't think I would ever be posted there. The Congo was colonised by Belgium until 1960, so the operational language is French. Humanitarian workers in the region communicate in French, translators translate from the local languages to French and all of the government meetings are conducted in French. I don't speak French, so I never imagined that I would work in the region.

Concern had a small team stationed in Goma, with an operational forward base in a town called Masisi, about eighty kilometres north-west. The development programs they ran were focused around livelihood, an area of humanitarian work devoted to helping people generate an income, but they also worked in rapid emergency response because of the rolling conflicts. The emergency work focused mostly around internally displaced people.

Different territories around Goma were controlled by different military groups, with battle fronts frequently moving around and impacting the local population. Rebel soldiers would move into an area, looting and pillaging, and the community would run away and end up in a new spot. Aid organisations would move in to help the displaced people to establish camps and to resupply the population with basic goods, and then when things calmed down the population would try to move back home. Things were constantly in flux in DRC, and Concern was one of many organisations that had established a base in-country to deal with the fallout.

The country manager was an Englishman named Toby. Before I was deployed to DRC, Toby had been working with other aid organisations in Goma to develop a new model for resupplying goods to displaced people. The standard model involved issuing something called a non-food item (NFI) kit stocked with essential goods such as blankets, jerry cans and cooking implements.

It was a basic start-up package for people who had nothing. But, as Toby had realised, the whole NFI kit wasn't always necessary. When people ran, they didn't run completely empty-handed, and when the soldiers looted villages, they didn't take everything away. When NFI kits were issued, people tended to end up with five blankets but no mattress, or five jerry cans but no spoon. A certain amount of the stuff we were giving out was effectively going to waste.

An organisation called CRS had come up with a model that used an artificial market to resupply internally displaced people. Traders would be invited to come and sell their goods at the market, which was only open to the refugee community. The refugees would be given vouchers that represented a certain amount of money and they could trade those vouchers for goods of their choice. At the end of the day, the traders would bring the organisation the vouchers they had collected and the organisation would transfer the equivalent amount of cash directly into their bank accounts. This system allowed people to purchase the goods they actually needed, with more security and controls than simple cash distribution would offer. In humanitarian aid terms, it was still considered a cash distribution program, but it was a lot safer than going door-to-door with envelopes full of money.

CRS had run the emergency response market four or five times in Goma and it had been very successful, so Toby wanted to try it in a more remote region. He wanted to roll it out in a place called Rubaya, a village halfway between Goma and Masisi with a large refugee population, and he needed an extra pair of hands. I was sent to DRC to help, though I had never run a cash program and I didn't speak the language. Toby also wanted to expand the project a bit. CRS had run markets for 200 families at a time. There were 5000 families in Rubaya.

The region around Rubaya was too insecure to base myself up there for weeks on end, so I was forced to drive up regularly from Goma to meet with the community—a four-hour round trip that I was making three or four times a week. Eventually, I got clearance to stay up there once or twice a week, but in the early planning phase of our market project, I spent countless hours on the road. There wasn't much I could do except listen to my iPod and watch the jungle slip by.

As the plan developed, I became more and more convinced that it was an excellent and very practical solution. We couldn't have given people cash and sent them off to a real market. There were no markets left in Rubaya because of the conflict in the area, so the only way for the community to access traders was if we brought them in. And because we controlled the market, we could control the prices for key items. There wasn't enough competition in the region to drive prices down, so traders could charge whatever they liked, which wasn't an efficient way for us to spend aid dollars. Instead, we would negotiate with traders to sell key items at a fixed price and allow them to bring in other goods—radios, batteries, fabric, et cetera—and set their own prices for those luxury items.

Because it was our market, we could also address other needs in the community. We discovered that people had stopped sending their children to school in Rubaya because no one could afford the fees, so we invited the school to participate in the market as well. The community could use their vouchers to pay the school fees in advance. We also invited agricultural traders in so that the community could buy seeds.

All of this had to be hashed out and explained to the community—the vouchers, the trade prices, the necessary goods and the luxury items, plus the system we would use to assess needs in the community and create beneficiary lists for the vouchers. The initial discussions took several days, purely because the concept was difficult to communicate. Again, I resorted to drawing pictures and comic strips to help explain the process. Again, the drawings got us over the line. Those drawing skills I'd picked up in South Sudan came in handy all the time.

Part of the initial planning phase involved establishing a relationship with the military group that occupied Rubaya, which was headed by a man known as Colonel Innocent. The colonel was a very refined man who spoke excellent English and French, always beautifully turned out in his army fatigues. He heard that we were looking for a base in Rubaya and offered us a house just outside the village.

Rubaya was beautiful, situated in a collection of lovely rolling hills with a river winding through them that made it look like the hobbit village in *Lord of the Rings*. The village was clustered on one side of the river. The colonel's house, three storeys high, was perched on top of a hill on the opposite bank. It was solid brick and the floors were made of cement, which made it a very lavish structure for this part of the world, but literally every window and door was either broken or missing.

On the day we went up to see the house, I sat outside with Colonel Innocent and drank tea. The colonel wore green army fatigues and a cream Ralph Lauren sweater, and a fedora with a large feather in the band. As we talked, he removed his boots to reveal purple Winnie the Pooh socks that had individual sections for each of his toes. *This man commands a rebel group that is probably responsible for raping and pillaging other villages in DRC*, I thought. Also, I didn't know they made toe socks for adults.

Colonel Innocent explained to me that the house was where he'd lived before the war. He had been a cheesemaker, which is why his home was three storeys high; the bottom floor was a cheese cave. He'd been a simple farmer back then, living a simple life. His dairy cattle had roamed the hill leading down to the river and drank water from its banks.

The colonel was very proud of his house and he was keen for us to use it, but it would have involved Concern carrying out the necessary renovations. We'd then be paying rent to someone who was part of the conflict. He was being very kind in offering us accommodation but I had to be equally kind in refusing him.

We cast our net a bit wider and found an old Christian refectory about thirty minutes outside Rubaya where we were able to set up our local base. The building was solid brick, but again, the windows were mostly broken. There was a toilet but it didn't flush because there was no running water. There were enough rooms to house the entire team, however. That was all we really needed.

Goma was a weird city. I had never seen anything like it. The long-term instability in the area had drawn a large cadre of humanitarian organisations to the town—everyone from the Red Cross and MSF to little indie organisations no one had ever heard of. The UN presided over the whole cluster, giving us daily security briefings and encouraging collaboration between different organisations. And because we all worked so closely together, the whole expat community felt like a scene.

I had, up until this point, managed to avoid the humanitarian aid cliché of working hard and partying even harder. There are whole books devoted to the boozy, sexually promiscuous lifestyle that so often accompanies major humanitarian interventions, but I had been too busy or too isolated in my work to really participate. Banda Aceh was probably my best opportunity, but the region was under Sharia law so all the expat parties were confined to people's houses, the booze was snuck in and people had to be discreet. I was also working twelve-to-fifteen-hour days in Aceh, under a huge amount of pressure. I couldn't afford the hangovers. In Goma, it was a different story. I worked long days and travelled frequently up to Rubaya, but at the end of the day the whole expat community in Goma cut loose. I did my best to keep up.

There were a bunch of restaurants down on Lake Kivu where all the foreign aid workers would converge every night, places like Coco Jamba where they served raw meat and we barbecued it at the table. We drank cold beer with dinner and then headed to one of three discos on the main street and drank some more. People got very messy. And while it was bigger than what I was used to, it was still a relatively small community. There was plenty of gossip circulating about who was sleeping with whom, who wanted to go out with whom, and who had broken whom else's heart. It was all fairly ridiculous.

I think people who worked in Goma needed to distract themselves from how unsafe it was. If you thought too hard about it, you probably wouldn't stick around. We often heard stories of lucky escapes and near misses, like the time an aid team from the US was held at gunpoint and forced to lie face-down in the dirt while their car was raided (though they were out for dinner and drinks that same night). On top of the security issues, the volcano looming over the city had erupted in very recent memory and the beautiful Lake Kivu was an overture lake, meaning it sat on a bubble of methane. If the bubble ruptured, it would cause a tsunami and the methane leak would kill everyone who hadn't drowned in the wave. This was something that could happen at any time, as far as we knew. Between the bullets and the lava and

the possible toxic poisoning, I guess we all had very good reasons
to drink.

One of the biggest tasks in putting the market together was creating
a beneficiary list. We needed to make a record of everyone in the
village who would qualify for vouchers, to create some kind of
framework for assessing who needed the most help. As we started
the research, it became clear that everyone in Rubaya had been
displaced multiple times and was essentially in the same position,
all with very high need. In the end, it became clear that we would
have to take 95 per cent of the population into the program—
pretty much anyone who wasn't working for the government or
the military.

The assessment work took time and involved frequent trips
up to Rubaya over precarious muddy roads. Our LandCruiser
had to work pretty hard to navigate the sludge and potholes,
and we were frequently stopped for hours at a time while other
vehicles were rescued from boggy ditches. There was a particular mountain pass just outside the village that seemed to get
worse over time, until we arrived one day to find that the road
had collapsed completely. It was suddenly less of a road and
more of a crater on the edge of a cliff. We had to enlist an army
of locals with picks and shovels to try to hammer it back into
shape. While this operation was underway, a team from MSF
arrived, on their way up to Rubaya for one of their twice-
weekly clinics. They insisted that they could make it through
the crater and told us all to stand aside. I warned them not to try
it, but they weren't interested in taking my advice. We all moved
aside and watched as their car struggled over the collapsed road
and their rear tyre slipped off the edge of the mountain. When
the second rear tyre slipped off the road, we thought they were

done for, but they had just enough speed to pull the vehicle back onto the road and up the other side.

'That's it, we're not crossing here anymore,' I said.

From then on, we made the journey with a system of 'kisses', where one car would drive us up from Goma and deposit us at the crater and a second car from Rubaya would be waiting to collect us on the other side. I wish I could say that was the end of our trouble on the roads.

One day, while travelling in a LandCruiser along a very straight piece of highway on our way to Rubaya, we saw a *mutatu* in the distance, coming towards us. *Mutatus* are small buses used throughout Africa as a form of public transport—twenty-seat vehicles that are always jam-packed with passengers and painted in wild, bright colours. The conductor would sometimes sit in the window, calling people to the bus and selling them tickets before they boarded.

The *mutatu* we saw out on the highway must have been doing more than a hundred kilometres an hour, but the conductor was still sitting in the window, with all but his legs and feet hanging outside the bus. As we watched, the *mutatu* driver lost control and the vehicle began to wobble. 'Stop, stop, stop,' I told our driver, though we were at least 600 metres away. We ground to a halt just as the bus started to flip. We could only watch as it turned lengthways and tumbled along the highway, spinning three times before it came to rest.

There was glass everywhere. The *mutatu* had been loaded with used glass bottles destined for a recycling plant in Goma, and they'd burst into a million shards when the bus had crashed. There was also a significant petrol leak running out of the tank, so I asked our driver to stop at a distance when we drove up to assess the damage.

I had a first-aid kit and fifteen local staff with me, only one of whom spoke English. There were twenty-three crash victims altogether, including the guy who had been sitting out of the window and who was now trapped under the *mutatu*. All of the skin had been grated from the back of his torso and skull, yet somehow he was conscious.

I raced back to the car. There was a lift jack on the top of our car and we needed it to move the bus safely, but I had no way of communicating what I was doing. I started unbolting the jack, then looked back to realise that four or five members of my team were trying to flip the bus. 'No, no, don't do it!' I yelled, scrambling back down off the car. I needed to manage the conductor's spine at the very least, he could bleed out, but they were using brute force to right the bus and get him loose. Meanwhile, the man's legs were still trapped inside the *mutatu*. When they flipped the bus upright, he went up with it, his body dangling out of the window. I dropped the jack and bolted to him, trying to support his head. The best we could do was drag him out and lay him down on the broken glass.

We managed to triage and move seventeen people in under twelve minutes, putting the conductor and the worst impacted passengers into the Concern cars and sending them off to the hospital in Goma. Two UN peacekeeping trucks pulled up while this was going on, but the soldiers watched impassively. 'If you're not going to fucking help, you can fuck off,' I yelled angrily. And sure enough, the trucks pulled away.

Later, Toby asked if Concern was expected to pay the victims' medical bills. There was no public safety net for medical treatment in DRC, and because I had been the one to send the passengers to hospital, it was likely I would be expected to foot the bill. This was news to me. I'd just done what I had been trained to do as a nurse.

I loved the Concern team in DRC. Toby was an excellent manager, if a bit mad. He'd found some African wax print fabric covered in beer logos and had a suit made out of it, which he often wore to work. It looked incredible with his ginger hair. Up in Masisi, there was a young Canadian woman named Cara and a Tunisian-born Englishman named Alec, who were both great fun and really good at their jobs. In Goma was a French guy called Theo who was, in my experience, typically French. He appreciated the local nightlife and was very much appreciated by the expat ladies. Theo lived by himself but kept a couple of rooms spare for Cara and Alec when they were in town, and I lived in another compound with Toby. We had an amazing cook, which was a new experience for me. One of the previous country managers had spent a lot of time teaching the cook French recipes, so we ate like kings—except on Christmas Day, when he had the day off. Cara and I decided to cook for the Concern team at Christmas, and we ended up with seventeen orphans from other aid organisations in Goma. We also picked up a new housemate.

When we had gone out to do the Christmas food shopping, Cara had found a kitten inside a hole in a besser-block fence and brought it home. It was only a few days old, very weak, but Cara was determined that I save it with my paediatric nursing skills. The poor thing had a pathetic little cough and we thought it might have pneumonia, so we spent a good part of Christmas Day trying to calculate the correct antibiotic dose for a patient weighing 300 grams. We had to feed it infant formula with a syringe every few hours to keep it alive, and the whole Concern team was drawn into the drama. I tried to tell Cara that we were just prolonging its suffering, but she wouldn't listen. She named the cat Heba. Alec decided that it was going to kill the rats in their house in Masisi.

When New Year's Eve rolled around, we were still nursing the sick kitten. It wouldn't have been a problem, but we were heading to a party at a hotel in Rwanda to avoid the 11 p.m. curfew in Goma. We had to smuggle the cat over the border in a box covered in some blankets, and while everyone drank themselves to oblivion that evening, we somehow managed to keep nursing the kitten. We had alarms set on our phones and every few hours, when the beeping started, someone stumbled off to feed her. We all slept on the beach that night and woke up huddled around the little fur ball.

Heba survived. She went up to Masisi with Cara and Alec and lived there for the next eighteen months and when Cara finished her mission, she brought Heba home. Heba now lives a very fancy life in Canada with Cara's mother, and I get regular photo updates, reminding me that I had wanted to put her out of her misery.

As the market date drew closer, I moved from Goma up to the refectory where the Concern team was based. One morning, I had to drive up to the collapsed section of the road to meet a car that was carrying the freshly printed market vouchers up from Goma. Our plan was to spend the next two or three days distributing the vouchers while the local army worked to repair the road, allowing the traders to arrive with their trucks just in time for the event.

The car from Goma was driven by a wonderful local guy called George, who was expecting a new baby with his third wife. George was sixty-five years old. He didn't speak English, but we did our best with the handful of French words I had collected and a lot of hand gestures. When I walked across the crater to meet him that morning, George was extremely agitated, though

I couldn't figure out why. In English, he told me, 'They're coming, they're coming.'

I had to get Toby on the radio to speak with George and figure out what was going on. Toby spoke to him and then to me again. 'He says the Rwandan army is coming. The Rwandan army is on its way.'

'What? What does that mean?' I answered.

'I'm not sure, but stay put—I'll find out and call you back.'

We were deep into DRC, nowhere near the Rwandan border. I was sure George must be confused. Then all of a sudden, I saw a soldier coming around a bend in the road. Then I saw three soldiers. Then I saw five. I stepped out into the road to get a better look and sure enough, there was a line of soldiers as far as I could see, marching single file like a column of ants.

It was obvious that this was a serious operation. Every fifth guy was carrying a case of food on his head; every twentieth guy was carrying a small generator. They all had guns. My first instinct was to jump on the radio and speak to Toby, but George caught my hand as I reached for it and shook his head. We watched silently as the entire platoon filed past, in matching bone-coloured army fatigues with a Rwandan flag patch on their shoulders. *Fuck. The Rwandan army is* here.

The history of the conflict was complicated, but one of the rebel groups operating in eastern DRC was the Federation for the Liberation of Rwanda (or FDLR, based on its original French name). The FDLR was made up of escaped Hutus who had been responsible for the Rwandan genocide, and the Rwandan army had entered DRC in the past on the pretext of hunting for these war criminals. But eastern DRC was also a mineral-rich area and it was suspected that the Rwandans had ulterior motives: they wanted to seize control of valuable natural resources. The

Congolese government had already fought a war to eject the Rwandan army, so it wasn't good news that it was back.

When the soldiers had disappeared around the next bend, I called Toby.

'The Rwandans crossed the border last night,' he told me.

'I know. I just saw them.'

'You need to come back. The market is off.'

'We can't call it off now, Toby! It's so close. We've told the community we're distributing the vouchers today, just let me tell them the plan has changed.'

'You've got one hour,' he told me. 'Then I need you to get into a car and get back to Goma.'

I took the vouchers from George and went back to meet the driver waiting for me on the Rubaya side of the crater. He had seen the platoon file past and was just as agitated as George, but I convinced him to get in the car and go. On the return journey to Rubaya, we passed the column of soldiers trudging along the road. I saw them, and they saw me, for a second time. I was a white woman in the middle of nowhere, so naturally I caught their attention.

I arrived back at the refectory and pulled everyone together. We decided that the army would travel into Rubaya by the walking track that cut through the mountains, not by the road. It should take them at least two hours to reach the village, which gave us just enough time to drive in and let the community leaders know what was happening. We wouldn't distribute the vouchers today, but the market was definitely going ahead and they shouldn't worry.

On the road into Rubaya, we saw the last of the Rwandan soldiers as they were leaving the road and heading onto the walking track. And yet again, they saw me. In town, the Concern team split up to reach as much of the community as quickly as possible. I gave them twenty minutes to get the word out, then we would rendezvous back at the cars and leave. I set out alone to find Colonel Innocent and the senior leadership team in the village, carrying with me all the gear I needed to pull out—my runaway bag on my back, the satellite phone, radio and camera clipped to my utility belt, and my mobile phone in my pocket.

I knew Rubaya very well by then, so I walked confidently through the winding streets that led to the centre of the village. I found one of the senior leaders drinking tea in his home. It was still very early in the morning. There was no phone signal in Rubaya, so I asked him to head up into the mountains once a day to get a signal so that we could call and update him on plans for the market.

By the end of our conversation, I realised that I had three minutes to get back to the rendezvous point, so I raced back through the winding village streets. Emerging from a laneway between two houses, I ran smack bang into the head of the Rwandan army line. They'd moved a lot faster than we anticipated. I stopped dead and watched them file past again, and for a fourth time that day the soldiers registered a strange white woman in their path. The column looked incredible, snaking over the nearby hills. I reached for the camera on my belt, thinking it would make an incredible photo, but something stopped me. *Not a good idea.* It wasn't that I was afraid, necessarily. We just had to be cautious until we understood what was going on.

I continued to make my way towards the rendezvous point. I was still alone but I could see the Concern car; I was virtually in spitting distance. As I walked, a Rwandan soldier fell in beside me and started talking to me in French. He seemed quite relaxed and polite, so I did my best to respond, smiling and nodding, though I didn't understand much of what he was saying. He reached down as we walked and held my hand, which wasn't all that alarming. African men are quite physically affectionate. Friends often held hands. I continued to smile and swung his arm a little as we walked. It had been quite an exciting morning—*the Rwandan army is here!*

When we arrived at the Concern car, the soldier sat down on a log, so I sat beside him. My translator arrived and walked straight over to us, speaking to the soldier in French. Not understanding the words, all I could do was read their body language, which very quickly told me something was wrong. The translator looked distressed. *Things are not okay.* I tried to stand up but the soldier put a hand on my shoulder and forced me down again. *Things are definitely not okay.*

'You've been arrested,' the translator told me. 'They think you are a spy.'

I started laughing, which was a mistake. The soldier's face hardened as if to say *this is not a joke*, but all I could think was that I must be the worst fucking spy in history. I didn't speak the language, I was six foot two, blonde, white and a woman. I stuck out like a grain of rice in a coffee jar; the whole thing was ridiculous. However, the soldier didn't seem to share my sense of humour.

A commander arrived and demanded to see my phone, the satellite phone and my camera. They thought I had been recording their movements throughout the day, taking photos of them and their position. Thankfully, there was nothing on the camera except photos of the village and the community members. I had spoken to Toby on the radio, so there was no call history on my phone or the satellite phone.

Colonel Innocent arrived just as the army finished going through my things and spoke at length to the commander. I sat quietly on the log and observed, but their body language didn't reveal much. It seemed cordial. Finally, the colonel walked over and pulled me to my feet, handing me my belongings. 'The army will be here for a few days,' he said. 'Please stay in contact with me. I will let you know when you are safe to return.'

That was the end of my Jason Bourne moment. It lasted about fifteen minutes.

Ultimately, we decided to hold the market while the Rwandan army was stationed in Rubaya. They had established a front to the north of Rubaya and were negotiating with a rebel group up near Masisi for the handover of some suspected war criminals, with a deadline of eight days before they escalated the conflict. Things would be relatively stable in Rubaya during that eight-day window, but there was no telling what would happen after the deadline. We decided to hold the market while we still could.

We were obviously concerned that we would distribute a whole lot of goods only for the village to be raided again, but Rubaya was in a relatively strong position. Colonel Innocent was allied with the Rwandan army, so Rubaya was actually more secure than it had been previously. More pressing for us was the fact that the villagers were in serious need of help. It was very cold up in the mountains, food was scarce and a lack of provisions could quickly escalate to a crisis.

From beginning to end, the market planning had taken six weeks but we were in a great position to roll it out. Cara and Alec had been evacuated from Masisi and were there to lend a hand, and the woman who was destined to replace me in DRC had arrived for the handover period, so we were very well staffed for the event. It was going to be a walk in the park.

We revised the model a little. Instead of handing out the vouchers in the village, we gave out tickets that would be exchanged at the market entry for the cash vouchers. No one had identification, so we had to go through a painstaking process of matching people by name to the beneficiary list, but this bought the traders some extra time to assemble their goods in Goma and gave the local army time to finish reconstructing the road. When the tickets were handed out, we were ready to roll and the trucks started coming in.

The market was set up on a small patch of flat ground down by the river. We roped off an area roughly half the size of a football field and planted two sticks in the ground to serve as a gate, with a Concern Worldwide banner mounted overhead. The stalls were arranged around the edge of the field, with the goods laid out on squares of tarpaulin, and the Concern team was stationed at the entry point to distribute vouchers and control the flow of traffic. We hadn't found a trader with decent quality blankets, so Concern had provided two blankets per household. When the market opened, I was sitting on a stack of blankets in the middle of the field, waiting to hand them out.

It worked beautifully. The villagers understood the system well and we had plenty of staff on hand to answer questions, all wearing high-vis vests with a Concern logo on the back. There were hundreds of women from the village, dressed up for the occasion in brightly coloured prints, and the atmosphere was joyful.

At some point on that first day, I was called to the entry point because a lady had turned up without a ticket, insisting she was on the list. When I arrived, I found the woman holding a newborn baby in her arms. By newborn, I mean hours old; it was still covered in birthing fluid. The woman told me she had missed out on collecting her ticket because she had been in labour. 'When did she have this baby?' I asked.

'When the sun got up,' the team told me. It wasn't lunchtime yet and the market was a good hour's walk from the far side of the village. The woman had given birth and then carried her child to the market because she was afraid she would miss out.

I took the baby from the mother to do a quick health check and told the team at the gate to give the woman her vouchers. She was incredibly grateful. She wanted to buy new fabric at the market to wrap her child in.

The first day of the market closed without a hitch, but later that evening I started to cough. As the night went on, I developed a fever. By morning, I couldn't walk and talk at the same time and I was struggling to breathe. It was clear I had a chest infection, so I couldn't go near the refugee population. I couldn't return to Goma, either, because we didn't have enough vehicles, so I sent the team to run the second day of the market and I stayed in bed at the refectory.

When the team came back at the end of the day, it was clear that things hadn't gone well. There had been tension between Cara and my replacement over who was in charge, and spot fires that they had struggled to deal with, so we decided I should be there on the third day to keep things under control. I felt marginally better, and all I really had to do was sit next to a pile of blankets. I stayed put in my chair and people came to me with problems, which I largely solved by radio. My favourite part of the whole day was watching women from the village shopping for new fabric, which they may not have done in years, unfolding and refolding bright bolts of colour as the day slowly faded away.

We ran the market for five days, servicing about 1000 people a day. It was a clear success and the whole team was very satisfied, as were the community and the traders. Back in Goma, the traders turned in their vouchers and we wired the payments, and then I checked myself into hospital because the chest infection still hadn't cleared up. It turned out I had pneumonia and something else. The doctors thought it may have been whooping cough. I remembered that I had been holding the newborn baby just before my symptoms developed, which means I would have been infectious at the time.

I called the MSF team working in Rubaya to let them know about the diagnosis and they told me they had already seen a few cases up in the village. In all likelihood, that's where I got it. In any case, they would follow up.

I had been vaccinated for whooping cough, so it didn't really make sense, but I was sick for weeks. I felt terrible; really guilty, despite all the good work we had done. Weirdly, the cough never went away completely. I still have the ghost of it, to this day.

# 14

# You'll have to google it

When Cyclone Larry hit the Queensland coast at Innisfail, I saw the best and worst of Australia. The whole country mobilised to respond to the disaster. The Queensland government did incredibly well with early warnings and preparedness in the lead-up to the storm, and money came pouring in to support the relief effort after it landed. Plane-loads of carpenters and tradespeople flew up to Queensland to help rebuild, and the community kicked into action to resupply people who were affected. The Australian government released emergency relief money through the social security system virtually the next day. But at the same time, there were people all over the nightly news complaining that they had no power or water.

Larry was a severe tropical storm, a Category 5. People in the developed world tend to have an expectation that their communities are disaster-proof, but it was incredible that anything was left standing at all. The definition of a disaster is that a community's resources have been overwhelmed. By definition, you're going to be without resources for a while. All along the Queensland coast, power stations were bent literally in half, just a mass of crumpled steel. And yet people were bitching about not having cold drinks.

If the same cyclone had hit the Philippines, thousands of people would have died. It could take us weeks to set up cash transfer systems to distribute relief funds in that context and years for a community to build back. Australia seemed to have no sense of its own privilege and it kind of pissed me off.

In 2009, I was sent for a short mission in Indonesia following the Sumatra earthquake. It was a 7.6 on the Richter scale and more than 1000 people had died—the perfect example of what a disaster can look like when a community is truly vulnerable.

Concern was working with a number of partner organisations in the region, most of whom were doing long-term development work in the aftermath of the tsunami. When the earthquake hit, the development teams quickly moved resources into Sumatra to respond to the crisis, but they asked for some additional emergency support as it wasn't necessarily their field of expertise.

I flew into Sumatra with Eric, the engineer on Concern's Emergency Response Team, two days after the earthquake—the earliest I had arrived in the wake of a major disaster. I wanted that experience purely because I hadn't had it yet. From my point of view, while there was important work to be done, it was also a professional development opportunity. This was old hat for Eric, and there was plenty I could learn from him during the deployment.

We were embedded with a team of very young Indonesian aid workers. They collected us from the airport and took us to our hotel in Padang, but Eric took one look at the place and refused to check in. 'It's not safe,' he declared. The earthquake had split the building in two: a perfect crack ran from the ground floor right up to the roof. Instead, one of our local team members took us to her mother's house. For a few days at least, we would sleep in her mother's guest room and eat meals with her family.

In addition to the aid organisations that had moved into Padang, the Australian military was in town. They had been doing tactical training near Sumatra and had quickly redirected their resources to the earthquake response. Despite the congestion, it was all running very smoothly, primarily because the Indonesian government had learned a lot from the tsunami. A cluster system had already developed and the response effort was well coordinated.

In Padang, we were mostly looking at structural damage. The landscape was littered with collapsed or crushed buildings that would appear suddenly whenever you turned a corner. Major multi-storey government buildings, built with cheap materials to poor safety standards, had fractured or folded in on themselves, shaken into unsteady pieces. But life in the Sumatran capital was already moving again. Many of the shops were still closed but stalls had begun to appear on the roadsides, and everywhere you looked people were clearing debris or cleaning. People weren't sitting around waiting for aid agencies to come and save them; they were busy trying to save themselves.

The most difficult thing in this scenario is trying to get an overview of what is happening; to understand the chain of command and find out what efforts are already underway, and then figure out where there are gaps that need to be filled. No matter where you are in a disaster response, you will come across some crisis that needs to be dealt with, but you are unlikely to know what crisis is happening in the next block or the next village. For Eric and me, the job in Sumatra involved finding command and control and figuring out how we could actually help.

Meetings—that's the first thing you do in disaster response. The search and rescue teams deploy immediately and the hospital teams roll out emergency services, but Eric and I spent the first two days in Padang trying to figure out what information people already had and what information was missing in order to formulate a plan about how to deploy our own resources. By this stage of my career, I was plugged into a network of technological resources that made disaster response much more efficient. I got text messages from the GDAC (Global Disaster Alert Coordination) system whenever there was an earthquake over a certain size, with information about the likely impact zone. We got satellite photos from the military and footage from media outlets, and paired it with information from disaster victims who were calling in to government and emergency services to build a picture of the overall impact. And when we didn't get calls from a particular area, we knew there was a problem.

One of those information black spots in Sumatra was up in the mountains. An aerial assessment had been done of the rural areas outside Padang, showing extensive damage, but there was very little information trickling down to the city. It was clear that whole villages in the mountains had been wiped out, obliterated by landslides, but no one had been up there to take a closer look.

Eric and I headed out with the local team, over roads that were still cluttered with debris and had sometimes fallen away altogether. The landscape was strange and uneven, a community completely intact on one side of a mountain and a field of mud and rocks on the other side, where another community had been buried.

We sometimes hit roads that were impassable but we always met people walking down the mountain who told us what they had seen. We collected as much information from as many sources as possible to build a picture of the damage, always feeding it back into the emergency response cluster working out of Padang.

Eric and I had US$100,000 of discretionary funds to spend in Sumatra and we decided to channel it into a cash-for-work program up in the mountains. We would pay villagers to help with the recovery effort, clearing water and sanitation points, and congested agricultural land. The purpose was not simply to get the work done, but to provide victims of the earthquake with a livelihood that would support their own recovery. Eric and I designed the program and went out to meet with the local community to get them engaged, but as soon as the foundations were in place, we decided to move on.

We had planned to be in Sumatra for two to three months, but the emergency response was so well coordinated and there were so many other organisations already established in the area that we couldn't justify setting up a Concern office. Instead, we decided that it was best to channel our aid dollars into one of our partner organisations and hand the cash-for-work program over to them. We were in and out of Sumatra in just ten days, but ten days was all we needed.

On my way home from Indonesia, I got a message from my friend Emma, who was on an HIV mission in Bali. She would have the weekend off and planned to go diving—did I want to join her? I sure did. For four days, we dived the crystal-clear waters north of Bali, ate fantastic food and enjoyed the amazing wildlife. Then, on our way back to Denpasar, Emma suggested a spa day. I'd previously had a deeply traumatic experience with a masseuse in Singapore—way too intimate—so I really wasn't keen on the idea, but Emma insisted, so off we went for some enforced relaxation.

I was meant to fly out at the end of the day, but when we arrived back at the hotel I struggled to pack my bags. I really couldn't move at all, which amused Emma at first. 'This is what *relaxed* feels like, Amanda. I know it's a new feeling for you.'

'Maybe,' I complained. 'But my brain is now disconnected from the rest of my body.'

'That's the whole point,' she laughed.

When I arrived at Denpasar airport, I couldn't find my way into the departures area—I had to ask a security guard for help. By the time I got to the lounge, the fog had mutated into a pulsing headache and pain in my joints, so I gave Emma a call. She told me to take a teaspoon of cement and harden the fuck up. That's a direct quote.

I caught a plane back to mainland Indonesia then a connecting flight home to Australia, and along the way my headache transformed into a raging fever, sweats and nausea. My main concern was getting cavity-searched at the airport in Brisbane because I looked like a drug mule, but they very kindly waved me through. By the time I arrived at my house, I'd decided that I felt much better.

The following day, I went out with a friend from the tsunami operation in Banda Aceh. She was on leave from an extended mission in Papua New Guinea and keen to make the most of her time in Brisbane. I agreed to one drink. We went on a bender that lasted the better part of thirteen hours. I'm not kidding, we got home at four in the morning. I took her to the airport the next day and the fever and sweats descended again, along with knee pain and slight disorientation. 'You must be allergic to airports,' my friend laughed. 'This is your body telling you to stay home for a while.'

Back home, I took my temperature—39.8 degrees. I walked out of my bedroom and announced to my sister that I had malaria and was going to drive myself to the hospital. 'Are you sure? Do you want me to drive you?' she asked. Tears sprung from my eyes. 'You're crying!' she said. I really wasn't well.

'I am not crying! I can drive myself, I just need to get a malaria test done before I start the medication.'

I rocked up at the Royal Brisbane Hospital at ten on a Sunday morning. I hated going to triage. I never felt sick enough and I was sure the nurse would tell me to go and see the local GP. I explained to the triage nurse that I very likely had malaria. 'But I've been in five countries in the last four weeks,' I said. 'Kenya, Uganda, DRC, Sudan and Indonesia. So . . . could be anything.'

The nurse took my temperature, now 40.3 degrees, and then rushed away. When he came back, he had a team of people with him and they were all wearing face masks. They whisked me into a pressurised room, following the safety protocol for bird flu, though it was clear to me that that was not one of the options.

The tests came back negative for malaria. 'Oh, it'll be chikungunya then,' I told the doctor. He looked at me blankly. A few people I had met in Indonesia had been infected with it— another virus spread by mosquitos. 'Can you spell that for me?' he asked.

'You'll have to google it.'

A couple of hours later my temperature had climbed to 40.6 and I broke out in a red rash. I called the medical team back in. 'Okay, I don't have chikungunya, I have dengue.'

'Look, stop trying to diagnose yourself,' the nurse scolded me. 'Let the experts handle it.'

'Okay,' I shrugged. *Take your time.* I was now confident it was dengue and that I had picked it up sleeping in the guest room of my colleague's house in Padang.

I ended up staying in the infectious disease ward for six days, completely purple from the waist down and violently sick with dengue. The doctors debated giving me a blood transfusion and recommended I get into a different line of work. 'If you get dengue fever again, you could go into haemorrhagic shock. This career path could kill you.'

*It hasn't killed me yet.*

They told me to take it easy for a few months, but a couple of days after I left the hospital I decided I felt much better. My managers at Concern were quick to shut down any ideas of me returning to work, though; they told me to call them in three months. What was I going to do sitting on the couch for three whole months?! I decided to do what every other normal person does—tick off a few bucket list items.

I flew down to South Australia to go diving with Great White sharks. Fantastic idea, until I was actually on the boat, bobbing up and down in the middle of the ocean after three connecting flights and a very early start. I realised I felt like complete crap and perhaps this was not one of my greatest decisions. As the team was dropping the cage and throwing chum into the water to attract the sharks and the rest of the divers were getting ready to jump into the cage, I hung over the stern of the boat trying not to vomit. Eyes on the horizon. Suddenly, without a sound, a great white popped vertically out of the ocean about a metre away from me. It took a bit of tuna, looked me square in the eye then disappeared again under the water. *Maybe I do need a bit of a break*, I thought.

# 15

# GASTRO OR HEATSTROKE?

In an evaluation of the emergency response to the 2005 malnutrition crisis in Niger, Concern Worldwide concluded that its own response had been far too slow. There were stories of Concern team members stepping over malnourished children on their way into schools to deliver education programs, not recognising the indicators that a major food security emergency was already underway. As a result, the organisation reviewed its own training and assessment protocols to ensure that every program it ran, regardless of its focus, was malnutrition-aware. Concern didn't want to be caught by surprise again.

All of the indicators were pointing to another malnutrition crisis in Niger in 2010. The country director was a young economist named Steven who was convinced that we could prevent the crisis if we responded early enough with a system of food supply and cash transfers. He asked me to come to Niger to help develop a proposal for the project, adding a nutrition component to his economic intervention model.

The project Steven was working on was based on root cause analysis. Instead of waiting for the kids to get sick and then trying to treat them, it involved figuring out why the kids were getting sick in the first place and trying to stop this outcome earlier in the chain of events. In Niger, there had been massive crop failure due to drought, which meant that there wasn't enough food at a household level in certain parts of the country. While there was a food surplus in other parts of the country, the families at risk didn't have any money to buy it. At first, they would reduce their family's food intake to one meal a day to try to make it through the hunger season. Eventually, their supplies would run out and the kids would begin to starve.

Niamey is a baked city, split in two by the Niger River, that feels as though it would be swallowed by sand if its inhabitants weren't constantly sweeping it away. In minutes, a sandstorm can rise up over the desert and blanket the capital, fine grit blowing in under the doors and cracks in the windows, coating beds, tables, television sets; everything covered in dust. When I arrived in Niger, Steven took me out to see the dunes on the edge of town, on the south-western fringe of the Sahara. The sand appeared almost pink, while the sky over the sand dunes was pale, almost white, as if all the colour had faded in the heat. I thought of Alice Springs, with its burning reds and brilliant blue skies. No two deserts look exactly the same.

A few days after I landed in Niamey, the catastrophic 2010 earthquake hit Haiti and I got a call from Richard, my boss, asking if I could jump on a plane and head over there. More than 100,000 people were dead and millions were displaced. The whole international aid community was mobilising to respond and the Concern team was already stretched. Much as I was keen to go to Haiti because of the sheer magnitude of the disaster—when you work in foreign aid you want to be where the action is—I knew the Niger program would be in trouble if I left, and the food security data I was poring over did not look good. We had a window of opportunity to prepare for the malnutrition crisis and we had to take advantage of it. I was also concerned that we would end up being short-staffed in Niger, which is a French-speaking territory like Haiti. We would probably struggle to find French-speaking staff to take care of malnourished kids in the desert when they could be partying with two-thirds of the humanitarian world during the Haitian recovery effort. That was the reality of the situation, unfortunately: Haiti was what we call a CNN emergency—very high profile. Niger was less sexy but still critical. Richard and I agreed that I should stay in Niger and focus on getting that program up and running.

Of all the places I had worked internationally up until that point, Niger was probably the least secure. A few weeks before my arrival, a kidnapping attempt had been made against American expats in the town of Tahoua where we were due to be working, most likely by a Salifi-jihadist military group that operated in the area. Armed men had stormed a hotel and demanded that the concierge tell them where the Americans were, not realising that their targets were actually African-American—two black guys who were sitting in the lobby while this whole scene played out, and who managed to escape through the front door while the terrorists ransacked the hotel.

The security threats seemed largely targeted on American and French people, the former because of the military group's allegiance with Al Qaeda and the latter because of some controversial problems around uranium exports to France. The Concern team in Niger included an Aussie, an Irishwoman and a Brit, and none of our respective governments paid ransoms for hostages, so we were basically worthless targets there, thus thought to be reasonably safe. Our biggest concern was making sure that people actually knew where we were from. The gendarmerie, or local police, went to great pains to refer to us by nationality and I started getting around in a Wallabies jumper, just to reinforce the point.

I had, by this stage, completed hard security training with Concern, which was a big step up from the induction I'd had at Australian Red Cross basic training. During the program, we role-played a variety of security breach scenarios: kidnapping, being assaulted at checkpoints, violent altercations. For the first day and a half of the training, we were asked to plan a kidnapping of a real Concern country director, using maps and data available on the internet. It was a fascinating process, and I seemed to have quite the knack for it. In trying to think like a kidnapper, I figured out the various ways I could be vulnerable in the field. I learned where people might sit to watch me, how they could track my movements, when I was most vulnerable, and this in turn made me more aware of what I could do to protect myself. I learned not to fall into a routine, not to take the same route to work every day. I became more aware of suspiciously parked cars and high-rise buildings that might provide good vantage points. In restaurants, I learned to note the exits and always sit with my back to the wall with a view of the front door. Once I started seeing the world this way, I couldn't turn it off. Even now, when I go to a restaurant at home, I'm not comfortable unless I'm sitting in the right place.

Steven's proposal to deal with the malnutrition problem borrowed a cash-transfer model that had been trialled by the Concern team in Kenya—a way of transferring money around using a basic mobile phone. One of the issues in a lot of the developing countries where we worked was that people did not have access to banks. You needed identification and an address to open a bank account, and money to put in it, which was planets away from the reality of most of the people we were trying to help. There were also very few bank branches in remote rural Africa.

Mobile carriers in Kenya had cottoned on to this problem and developed a system called M-Pesa which allowed people to store money in their mobile account and transfer it via SMS. They used the M-Pesa system in Kenya like we use debit cards in Australia, but the system had yet to develop in Niger, and Steven was keen to get it up and running to facilitate cash transfers to people who needed aid. He had opened the conversation with local phone companies but wanted me to take it over, while at the same time establishing a malnutrition program that was a scaled-up version of the one we had run in Ethiopia.

The cash program was designed to stop families from using negative coping mechanisms—ways of adapting that had a gradually corrosive impact. Often when food ran out and there was no money, the young men in a family would leave to seek work in another country so that they could send money home. But it meant that those men weren't around for the next planting season, which would affect the following harvest. When they did come home after living abroad, they sometimes introduced HIV to their remote communities.

In a food security crisis, families would also sell off their assets, such as live animals or farming tools, just to buy food in the short term. They would eat the seeds that had been put away for the next planting season, out of desperation. And when the next season came around, they would have less than nothing. Multiple bad harvests could cause a total breakdown in food supply, which would lead to a major malnutrition crisis. Niger had already experienced a bad harvest in the preceding year and the ministry of agriculture had released a report predicting a 30 per cent crop yield with the coming harvest, so we knew trouble was on the way.

As in Ethiopia, 'malnutrition' was a dirty word in Niger. We had a major program to roll out and we needed buy-in from the government, but we had to talk around the real issue and be vague with our language. It didn't help that I couldn't speak French. I had a translator glued to me who became responsible for very high-level negotiations, and there were a number of very tense meetings as we battled through the opposition. The government insisted there wasn't really a problem in Niger, while we insisted that there would be.

At one particular meeting with the ministry of health, a doctor at the table who had been educated in English took me aside and said, 'Please keep going, we need this, but I can't say this out loud in the meeting. You have to find a way to convince them.' During the meeting, the doctor insisted that the hospitals and clinics in Niger had enough staff and training, and did not need additional support.

This meeting took place in Tahoua, a district in the far north. On the way back to Niamey we received a call from head office telling us to get off the road as there had been a coup d'état. We were advised to find the closest hotel and stay put. The local team huddled around the radio listening to the details of the coup as it unfolded, virtually a live broadcast of the events, but everything seemed to wind up just as quickly as it had started. Shortly after we had checked into the hotel, we got a call to let us know that the coup had been successful and that the military were in control of the government. We were safe to get back on the road.

Niger had a history of fairly peaceful coup d'états, one government seizing power after another. In this instance, the military leaders had decided that the government had misled the people and was not preparing properly for the malnutrition crisis ahead. As we left the hotel, I chatted with my local driver about it. 'That was quite efficient, really. Twelve minutes and only three people dead,' I noted.

'The last one was only eight minutes and one person dead, so this one is not as good.'

After the coup, the whole political dance around the malnutrition crisis evaporated. The military leadership made a public announcement and threw their full support behind our program. Within four hours of our very difficult meeting, the English-speaking doctor called me and said, 'Please come back, we are ready.'

The early intervention program was actually quite progressive, so we paired with a research specialist from Tufts University in Massachusetts in the US to set up a program that could be properly measured for useful academic data. If it worked and we could prove it, the model would be adopted much faster in future. We selected 7000 families to receive cash every month for five months, half via M-Pesa transfer, known as Zap in Niger, and half via brown envelopes. Another 3000 received a cash transfer at the beginning of the program and a second payment at the beginning of planting season, along with an allocation of seeds. Meanwhile, we scaled up the malnutrition program in Niger by adding staff into the ministry of health clinic and running nutrition training. We also added the CSB flour and oil as part of the supplementary food program to the existing Plumpy'Nut distribution.

The amount of cash we were distributing each month was adjusted based on the price of food in the market and we monitored the market to make sure enough food was coming in. The theory was that while food was scarce in Niger at that time, the influx of cash would help the market to maintain itself, whereas if people stopped spending money, the market would collapse. If the market collapsed, we'd have to change our program very quickly to food distribution.

The problem was so widespread in Niger that we couldn't reach everyone, so the government selected 116 villages that were very high risk. We accepted the recommendation wholesale, which was a bit unusual. Governments in this context are usually biased and unfair in their assessments, but Steven was convinced that the Nigeriens had been as objective as possible, so we took the list and tried to determine which families in those 116 villages would be selected for the program. Again, we couldn't reach everyone.

Early in the program, we visited a village where the corn stalks had grown high and the landscape was relatively green. *How can there be a food insecurity issue here?* I wondered. *There's food every-where.* But we crested a hill and the landscape on the other side was as barren as the moon. The rains had come, but only on one side of the hill. Three-quarters of the village had no food at all and a quarter had had a reasonable crop.

To develop our beneficiary list, we had to look for poverty indicators. It's difficult for people to be honest about how much they have if they are likely to be given something when they lie, so instead we relied on a study that had been done in Niger that showed relative wealth connected to assets. We knew families that did not own any animals were very poor. If they owned less than one goat or less than three chickens, they were a little poor. Middle-class people would have shoes but less than five goats, et cetera. Instead of asking people what situation they were in, we developed pictures of different families with differ-ent assets and asked people to self-select whichever picture was most like them. A certain level of pride kicked in when people were looking at the pictures, which made them unlikely to rank themselves lower than they actually were. In fact, as we discovered, people were more likely to move themselves up a class, which helped us to identify the truly ultra-poor people in the community who were in most need of help.

All through the process, we had researchers from Tufts checking and assessing our methodology to find out if people were satisfied. Those families that were brought into the program got quite a lot out of it, including mobile phones and cash, but no one ever complained that the system was unfair.

I pushed the team in Niger very hard to get the program set up because the spectre of Haiti was still looming. The scale of that disaster was becoming more and more apparent every day and I worried that I would get dragged out of Niger before we were up and running. Within weeks we were ready to roll, so I put out the call for reinforcements. I rang Cara and Alec, my colleagues from DRC, and essentially begged them to come help. We would put the 'old team' together again. It would be fun, I promised.

We were joined by a tiny Irishwoman named Anne, who was based in Niamey and married to a Nigerien man. Later we were joined by a young American intern called Andy who we nicknamed 'Pup' because he was just so excited to be helping out; he was like a puppy running in circles and peeing in the corner. We were nervous about having an American on the team because of the security issues it presented, but we were several months in by the time Andy arrived and our relationships with the local police felt strong enough to protect him.

Having a great team meant the difference between hell and a good time on a mission like that. We worked six and a half days a week in 45-degree heat. When we had time off it was too hot to go outside and too insecure to leave the house. When you live in such close quarters for months on end, tempers can flare easily, but the team in Niger got along well, and we found ways to keep ourselves occupied. Anne liked to meditate, but Alec, Andy and I preferred tennis—Nintendo Wii Tennis, in the safety of our living room. We played so much that I had to ice my shoulder every night, and I came home one Sunday evening to find Alec almost passed out on the couch with heat stroke. He'd been playing Wii all day in the air-conditioned house without drinking enough water. Our downtime was serious business.

The program was absolutely massive. We hired local agricultural experts to help with the seed distribution program, clinical staff to run the malnutrition clinic, and a group of women called the Mamma Lumias who we coopted from a breastfeeding program to run mobile phone training clinics and health promotion. The local team for the project sprawled to more than a hundred people.

We ran into trouble when it came to registering mobile phones for the thousands of women enrolled in the Zap part of the program because the women needed identification, though any ID would do. We decided that the best way forward was to photograph the women as we registered them and print our own identification cards. We taught the Mamma Lumias to use laptops and webcams out in the field to take headshots of the program participants—training sessions that literally started with *this is how you turn it on*. Within a week, thousands of images came back to us, which we then printed with an ID card machine I'd purchased online. The machine was fairly basic, designed for one card at a time, but we had it running day and night. It jammed often. As we got closer to the distribution deadline, Alec slept in the printing room, waking up whenever the machine ground to a halt to get our production line moving again. He aged ten years that week.

The biggest problem we encountered was the distribution of cash in envelopes. We had to divide roughly fifty thousand US dollars a week into $32 packets. Hundreds and hundreds of different envelopes had to be prepared and sorted. The local team advised that the women were far more trustworthy than the men, so the Mamma Lumias were nominated as the project's accountants. Every Monday, we locked the Mamma Lumias and Alec in a room at the local bank to count out and bag all the envelopes, then store the triple-checked packets in sealed bags and locked boxes. Each morning when it was time to do distribution runs, the teams would sign in at the bank, take two bags full of envelopes and transfer them to a locked box that was bolted into the back of their vehicle, then drive out to the village to distribute the cash to people with the correct identification card.

The operation ran very smoothly, but the gendarmerie was concerned that we were moving so much money so frequently along fairly predictable routes. We had to notify the villagers that the cash was coming a couple of days in advance because we needed them to be there to pick it up, but that was a lot of notice for anyone who might want to plan a robbery. The gendarmerie offered an armed guard to accompany the distribution teams and for the first time in my career, I thought it was wise to accept it. Concern didn't normally work with the armed forces, but in this case, after careful assessment, they decided to make an exception.

We distributed nearly half a million dollars during this operation and we only lost five dollars. A note blew away in the wind as it was being counted in a village. The team members were beside themselves. To my mind, *only* five dollars was a bloody miracle. I took it out of my pocket and added it back to the pile. Zero dollars lost!

The government announced halfway through the program that it was going to start distributing food rations to families on the beneficiaries list, which meant that certain families would be double-dipping in terms of emergency aid. We agreed to take on the food distribution on behalf of the government in order to manage the issue and ensure whatever resources were available were spread as efficiently as possible.

The handing out of the food was problematic for us, just because of the scale of the problem. There were massive numbers of people involved, especially in urban Tahoua. We tried to spread the load by running different distribution days in different parts of the city, but we realised quite quickly that people were moving with us, picking up food from multiple locations. We quickly determined that we would have to run distribution at every site simultaneously, which meant distributing food to 10,000 people on one single day.

The temperature in Niger soared to 49 degrees in the summer, a heat so crippling that it would cook your eyeballs if you took your sunglasses off outside, and we began to run into problems. The lines for food rations were incredibly long and people ran out of patience quickly, and we had a security incident at a distribution point inside the soccer field at Tahoua when the crowd surged. Three thousand women had arrived to collect rations and they were asked to move into a single line in order to enter the stadium, and the unhappy and overheated crowd began shoving and jostling against the metal turnstile gate. A woman was crushed, ending up in hospital with bruised ribs. In the end we asked the gendarmerie to provide guards, at least in Tahoua, to protect the food distribution program as well.

Between our cash and food programs, we had nineteen cars leaving the Concern headquarters every day, all heading off in different directions. Alec and I managed what we called 'school duty'. Every day, we would get up before sunrise to make sure the 'kids' all got to where they needed to be. It was chaos, every day, for months. Someone would arrive and then want to go and get breakfast, or the daily tea and milk rations wouldn't be equal and we'd have to sort it out, or some team member would be missing, or there would be some issues with the distribution lists. We had to get people into the right cars and heading off to the right place, and it always felt like we were their mums, getting them off to school.

One morning, when they were due to set off for a village we hadn't visited before, I got frustrated with a team that was horsing around and made the snap decision to jump in the car with them. 'Right, everyone, get in the car, it's time to go.'

I didn't mind heading out with them. Being with the community was my favourite part of the job—it made the long hours at the desk answering emails and working on budgets actually mean something. Besides, I was coming to the end of my placement in Niger. I wanted to see the program in action while I could. I grabbed five litres of filtered water in a portable can, let Steven know where I was going and set off for a small village in northern Niger. The village was inhabited by people from the Tuareg tribe, part of a semi-nomadic Muslim ethnic group that lives in and around the Sahara, and is famous for the dark indigo robes and face paint worn by the tribeswomen. There were thousands of women gathered when we arrived, with ornate head wraps and turquoise jewellery, and dark robes hanging dead straight to the ground in the 40-degree heat.

We were late and the scene was chaotic, and there was little I could do to communicate with the tribespeople because neither they nor I spoke French. My instructions were translated twice before they got to the intended recipients, and all I could do was hope that what they heard made sense. We made a plan, and I left the local team to the organisation and negotiations and instead started hauling 25-kilogram bags of food off the back of our truck.

Within a couple of hours, we had distributed nearly one and a half tonnes of food and I had drunk all five litres of water that I'd brought with me. Each of our cars carried forty litres of water in jerry cans in case of emergencies. I was faced with a dilemma that I normally tried to avoid at all costs. The water in the jerry cans came from the taps at our office in Tahoua and, for me at least, it wasn't safe to drink. I eyed the water suspiciously. It was so unbelievably hot that I wasn't even sweating anymore. That wasn't a good sign. *Gastro or heatstroke? Gastro or heatstroke?* I debated. I decided that heatstroke was inevitable if I didn't drink but I had a fifty-fifty chance when it came to the gastro. I would have to roll the dice and hope I didn't end up spending the next three days on the toilet. I helped myself to about six litres of the very turbid and unsavoury-looking water and crossed my fingers.

Part way through the mission in Niger, I had flown to Dublin for the semi-annual meeting of Concern's emergency team. I'd decided to take a little extra time to do a short course in infectious diseases at the London School of Hygiene, leaving Alec to manage the Niger program in my absence. I was only meant to be in London for a week, but the Eyjafjallajökull volcano had erupted in Iceland while I was there, spewing a huge cloud of toxic dust over Europe. I'd found myself grounded with time to kill and a new friend I'd met during the course. A— was an epidemiologist with a background in microbiology who was working for the Centre for Disease Control and Prevention on an HIV program in the DRC. We only spent a few days together, but there was a genuine connection and when I returned to Niger, A— called me every day. We usually exchanged texts right after I'd gotten the 'kids' off to 'school'.

When I made the snap decision to go to the Tuareg village, I had forgotten to let A— know and my mobile phone reception quickly dropped out. I was in radio contact with Steven, which was the most important thing. On the way back to town, the coverage kicked in again and I got a flurry of text messages from A—. The first said, *Where are you? I haven't heard from you today.* The second said, *Why aren't you answering me?* The third said, *I'm starting to get worried. If you don't answer me in the next half an hour, I'm calling someone.* The final, somewhat sheepish text message said, *I called your boss. I'm really sorry.*

In a panic, A— had googled Steven's telephone number and contacted him to tell him I might have been kidnapped, and Steven had gently let A— know that I was and had always been fine. I had been out of phone contact for less than six hours. I didn't know if I should be mortified or flattered. I guess it was a bit of both.

I was not going to get away clean. In the days leading up to my departure from Niger, the jerry can water that I had drunk while out in the Tuareg village finally caught up with me. I had the worst gastro of my life—and I had had some fairly horrific gastro. After two days of moaning and sweating on the couch, Anne forced me to go to the hospital, promising me I had nothing to worry about as it was the best hospital in Niger. *Whatever.* Niger was the poorest country in the world, and the best hospital in the poorest country was still less than average. I was sick enough to go there anyway. I walked through the reception doors, dramatically projectile-vomited across the waiting room floor, and keeled over in a dead faint. I spent three days in hospital, missed a flight for a holiday rendezvous with A—, and the doctor told me that my faecal specimen was pretty much entirely pus. He was quite impressed.

Despite the gastro, I was very happy with the way the mission turned out. The program that we created in Niger was quite complicated. We were monitoring markets as well as malnutrition rates, adjusting the cash distribution accordingly, adapting beneficiary lists and running massive, regular food distribution. Ultimately, it was too difficult to recruit someone with both cash experience and malnutrition experience who could also do the program analysis, so I stayed in Niger until the peak of the crisis had passed. I was meant to be in-country for six months, but the mission had sprawled out to nearly eleven months by the time I handed things over to Alec.

I loved the project in Niger because it was a large and complex thing to manage, and it was a new way of tackling a recurring problem that turned out to be very successful. The research showed very clearly that we had prevented a malnutrition crisis, with the global malnutrition rates staying well below normal, let alone reaching crisis levels.

Because I was preoccupied, I never made it to Haiti. I am one of the few people in the humanitarian world that didn't, it seems. For the rest of my career, Haiti was a major reference point for everyone in the industry and I got quite sick of hearing about it, to be honest. When I started running training programs later in my career, I developed a zero tolerance policy. If anyone started a sentence with the words 'But, in Haiti . . .' I made them put twenty cents in a jar.

# 16

# WE'RE GOING TO NEED A
# BIGGER CHAINSAW

In 2010, Ivory Coast president Laurent Gbagbo was accused of stealing an election. It was the first election held in the Ivory Coast in ten years and both Gbagbo and his opponent, Alassane Ouattara, claimed victory. When Gbagbo dug in and refused to cede power, Ouattara launched a military offensive to oust him and the Ivory Coast was thrown into conflict and unrest.

Ouattara's forces targeted Gbagbo's supporters in a bloody campaign, terrorising and torturing people as they moved to seize control of the country. The resistance crumbled and Gbagbo's supporters fled, creating a massive and rapid flood of refugees across the border into Liberia.

Just across the border, in a town called Ziah, Concern Worldwide was supporting an agricultural development program, providing guidance to the aid organisation that was responsible for program delivery. When refugees from the Ivory Coast started coming in, early in 2011, the local organisation asked for Concern's help to build a transit camp.

Transit camps are designed to give displaced people somewhere to rest on their way to a more permanent refugee camp. The United Nations High Commissioner for Refugees (UNHCR) had established a camp in the Liberian city of Zwedru and many of the Ivory Coast refugees had already made it there, but the rains were starting and there were more people on the move, already exhausted from the long walk out of danger.

When I arrived in Ziah, I found half a dozen tents erected on the football pitch in the middle of the village, already overcrowded. I was supposed to set up a medical checkpoint to assess which of the refugees were well enough to keep walking and which would need emergency care, and we planned to distribute food and oral rehydration salts, allowing people to rest for a day or two before they moved on. As usual, I was only meant to be there for a few weeks, but the mission quickly grew into something much bigger than we intended.

I was surprised to find that the people fleeing the Ivory Coast were largely middle class. There were politicians and protesters still wearing Gbagbo T-shirts, and many other professional people who were caught up in the conflict. They arrived with nothing but the clothes on their backs, but at home they were mechanics, teachers and shopkeepers, forced to flee purely because they had supported the wrong candidate. Some of the villages along the border had been attacked during the school day and the children had had to run, so mixed in with the rest there were many unaccompanied minors, still wearing their school uniforms.

They were lucky; the community in Ziah welcomed them with open arms. Many of the locals had fled across the border in the opposite direction during the recent Liberian civil war, and they were grateful for the aid they had received in the Ivory Coast. Some of the people coming back across the border now were actually Liberian by birth, and many others were connected to Ziah by family or friendship, and found people to take them in. The problem was that there were very few resources to go around. The local population had been so mobile during the civil war that they hadn't developed any kind of agriculture, even though the land around them was fertile, lush with thick jungle growth and green grass fields. There was no market in Ziah and barely any food. This is what the agricultural development program had been trying to address, but with the influx of refugees the town was completely overwhelmed.

The agriculture team had a five-year plan in the region and they had started building a couple of houses to hold their program staff. I was offered one of these houses as accommodation, though it was more of a shell than a house at the time. It had cement floors and walls, but no windows or running water. Again, I thought I would only be there for a couple of weeks, so camping on the floor seemed like a reasonable option.

Shortly after I landed, the agricultural program manager came down with malaria and was evacuated, leaving me as the only expat in Ziah. I then got a call from the Concern regional manager in Zwedru to let me know that the UNHCR refugee camp was full. The UNHCR had started work on another, larger site but had found unexploded ordnances buried in the ground and stopped construction. They wanted me to halt the flow of refugees from Ziah to Zwedru until they resolved the problem. There were roughly a hundred families in Ziah by this time, with twenty more arriving every day, and together Concern and the UNHCR had come up with a solution. The little transit camp, 5 kilometres from the Ivory Coast border, would transform into a full refugee camp.

Ironically, the UNHCR decided that Ziah was too insecure for its team, so I would remain the only expat in town, overseeing this transformation. My UN contact was an Australian engineer named Kate, who would come down once a week to check on the program, though she had to be back on the road to Zwedru well before dusk. Concern had made a different risk assessment and was already set up to operate in the area long term; the recent conflict hadn't changed that. The fact that my house had neither doors nor windows didn't really faze them.

If our plan to build a camp in the middle of the jungle was going to work, I would need help from the people who needed our aid, so we called a community meeting. This wasn't a cohesive community, really, just a ragtag bunch of people who had run from a bunch of different places, so I was surprised to learn that they had organised themselves into a functional hierarchy already. When I asked to speak to the community leaders, everyone knew who to send.

We held our first meeting in the backyard of a local house, while the owner's trained monkey danced on a lead in a very distracting way. One of the refugee community leaders pulled out a sheet of butcher's paper on which was drawn the most complex organisational chart I have ever seen. They had allocated ministries to each member of the leadership team: a minister for youth, a minister for women, even someone representing people with disabilities. Their committee structure was very horizontal, with two guys at the top and a bunch of sub-lieutenants with different fields of responsibility, including water, housing and education. I couldn't help but wonder if they had been 'developed' before, some time before this particular crisis.

When I told the committee we couldn't move and would have to stay in Ziah, they said, 'Okay, but these are the things we want.'

*Come again?* I thought. This was a bit unusual.

The committee gave me a long list of requests, starting with a request to activate the mobile phone tower on the edge of Ziah. The community didn't know where their families were or what was happening back in the Ivory Coast. They could listen to the BBC World Service on the radio, but it didn't tell them what was going on locally; as far as they knew, they may actually be able to go home. It sounded like a rich request, but I decided it was actually very practical.

The committee also requested a bus to take them into Zwedru once a week to do some shopping. The UNHCR would supply additional tents and food rations, but the community was missing basic items like toothbrushes and razors. Some of them had money to spend, if they could access a market. I wanted to laugh. 'I'm sorry, there are no buses,' I told them. 'Actually, there is hardly a road . . .' *How about I build you some toilets instead?* Later, some entrepreneurial people in Ziah started a motorcycle taxi service. It's always the way—the free market meets demand.

Their most optimistic request was for meat to be included in their food rations. The UN had already sent a shipment of bulgar wheat but no one knew how to cook it, including me. It also tasted kind of miserable. Could we get them a bit of animal protein the next time round? No, we couldn't supply meat, but I couldn't fault them for trying. No, we couldn't supply fish either, I apologised. *This is not a resort.*

I couldn't get the mobile phone tower turned on, despite my best efforts, and I felt terrible. It's one thing not to have phone reception, but if you're living right underneath the tower, it's like a quiet form of torture. Every day, I'd see people wandering around holding their phones up in the air, hoping against hope. We did manage to build toilets, however, and made sure everyone had somewhere to sleep within just a few days.

Within a few weeks, there were about 300 families living on the football field and another 200 living with family and friends in the village who received food rations from the UNHCR. In addition to building the infrastructure in the camp, we distributed materials to the host families so that they could build toilets near their homes, adding seventy-odd new facilities around Ziah and reinforcing the town's waterholes.

Eventually, we ran out of space to house people on the football pitch, and it didn't look like our displaced community would be moving anywhere soon. Kate and I agreed that we would need to build a formal refugee camp from the ground up, but where? The main problem was that we didn't have any land. Beyond the football pitch, there was virgin jungle, thick with trees and under-growth. The only way we were going to build a camp was if we cleared away a whole patch of jungle.

'I guess if that's what we have to do, we do it,' Kate said.

She went back to Zwedru to negotiate with the Liberian gov-ernment and then returned to Ziah with a GPS unit. I climbed into her LandCruiser and we set out on a dirt road towards the back of town, up a hill and into jungle so thick I couldn't see more than a couple of metres ahead. Our driver pulled out a machete and cut a path for us through the trees.

'Right, this is where we're building the camp,' Kate said, glancing at her GPS unit and pointing into the jungle. 'Five hundred metres that way and 200 metres that way.'

'You're fucking kidding,' I laughed. 'Where?' We were literally surrounded by trees.

'You'll have to cut it down,' Kate said. 'Can you do it?'

'I guess we don't have much choice.'

*I'm going to environmental hell*, I thought.

I hired a chainsaw team in the village and set them to work, ripping and growling through pristine jungle and burning off the waste. It was then time to get the refugee committee involved. I needed a labour force to help with clearing and construction, and since the community members were just sitting around, they were obviously the best option. We established a cash-for-work program to fund their labour, which pumped more aid dollars into the community and got everyone enthusiastic about the project.

Kate had created a schedule for the construction project that involved clearing 100 metres of land each week, but we had barely finished 20 metres when the first week elapsed. I went to meet with the committee to find out what the problem was and found half of them lying exhausted on the ground with blisters all over their hands. 'We don't usually do this kind of work,' they apologised.

'I am a hairdresser!' one women cried.

Another man said, 'I am a deejay!'

The middle-class refugee community was new to manual labour and I couldn't help but empathise. I liked gardening, but I wouldn't last more than two days doing nothing but pulling weeds. And we had still hundreds of metres to go. The community, to its credit, got jungle-slasher fit and the demolition continued at an exponential rate.

I lived on tinned tomatoes and tuna in Ziah, and continued to sleep on the floor of a house with no doors or windows. My bathroom was a bucket and a piece of tarpaulin wrapped around a couple of sticks, tucked away in the jungle behind the house. I'd have to get undressed inside the house, wrap myself in a towel and carry a bucket of water out the back, hang my towel on a tree branch and crouch down next to the tarp to wash myself. My 'shower curtain' was only a metre high and yet again mine was the only white arse for hundreds of kilometres.

One day, on my way back into the house after my daily crouch and wash, I felt a vicious bite on my stomach, then another one on my back. I yanked the towel away from my skin instinctively; sure enough, the towel was covered in bull ants, and I was covered in bites. *Motherfuckers.* I swore and hopped around in nothing but a pair of sneakers, and of course that was the moment some kids from the neighbourhood decided to walk past. Dignity, always just out of reach.

I caved after a few weeks and hired a French-speaking refugee named Angela as my cook, desperate for a little comfort, but it was still seriously rough living. I was covered in sawdust and grime pretty much all the time and my clothes really took a beating. The soles of my Blundstones melted when we were burning back the jungle—I felt the heat coming through the base of my feet and the boots sort of disintegrated after that. Meanwhile, I had managed to tear a massive hole in my one sturdy pair of jeans.

I had to visit Zwedru to buy replacement clothes from the second-hand traders, and ended up with an enormous pair of pre-loved hiking boots, which looked like they'd arrived direct from the Austrian highlands. Replacement jeans were a bit harder to come by, so the traders kept steering me towards their range of second-hand skirts. *No, thank you!* But the jeans they had were for skinny black men, not a white titan like me. The only pair I could find to fit me had diamante skulls on the back pockets.

We built up a good rhythm, cleared 100 metres of land in the jungle and put up tents and toilets, relocating the football pitch. Things were going so well that the UNHCR decided to start sending refugees back to Ziah from Zwedru. They were really stuck in Zwedru because they couldn't dig and they couldn't secure more land. 'Cut some trees down,' I teased Kate.

As more people arrived in Ziah and the camp expanded, I got increased support from Concern and the UNHCR. I was given a satellite beacon for internet, which meant I could order construction materials much more easily, and visitors came down from Zwedru a couple of times a week to supervise different elements of the project. It was all very social. We were ticking along and I was having a great time.

In the camp, life was flourishing. A few babies had been born and they had been named after me—middle names, I insisted, because Amanda is a very weird name to have in that part of the world. It was very cool, though. People had settled into their temporary homes, created little kitchens and set up market stalls to sell basic items they had picked up in Zwedru, so the camp was starting to feel like a small village. The progress made me happy.

We had even started a little hygiene program, building hand-washing stations called 'tippy taps' near the toilets. They were four-litre containers with holes in the lid, attached to a piece of rope that was in turn attached to a wooden lever. When you stepped on the lever, the container would flip over, water would pour out of the holes and you could wash your hands—a neat little bush solution when there was no running water.

One day, as I was doing my afternoon tour of the camp, I saw a young boy go into a toilet and then emerge again, walk over to the tippy tap and wash his hands. I felt a buzz of satisfaction—*our hygiene program is working!* Only a few weeks earlier, people had been defecating in among the construction debris. But my satisfaction turned to confusion as I saw the kid walk away from the tap with his pants still hanging down around his knees. *What is he doing?* I wondered. As I watched, the kid pulled his bum cheeks apart and wiped his bottom on a fallen log. *Oh christ*, I thought, *they don't have any toilet paper.* Pride could only last so long, as I discovered. There were always more problems to solve.

The community kept up their requests for meat but I wasn't able to provide it, so I was surprised to smell barbecue as I walked through the camp one afternoon. I found a bunch of people sitting around a fire, turning a spit roast of some unidentifiable animal. 'What is it?' I asked. 'Rats,' he said. 'Rats, from the jungle.' *Oh god.* People were so desperate they had resorted to eating vermin. 'Oh no,' they laughed. 'This is a delicacy, even at home.'

I wasn't tempted by the rat. I could live without meat, in fact I had to go out of my way to avoid it at times. One day when I was sitting on the front porch of my house, I saw a group of kids walking along the road pulling something behind them, something very small. The string went all the way to the ground, where it was attached to a small chameleon. 'Can I see it?' I asked. I picked up the little lizard and it was just amazing, eyes spinning nearly 180 degrees in their sockets, its feet like tiny hands. 'What are you going to do with it?' I asked.

'We're going to kill it!' the kids told me.

'What?!' I replied. 'No! You can't.'

I made a lazy Sunday afternoon mistake and gave them a dollar for the chameleon. I had no idea what to do with it, so I decided to keep it in a bucket overnight and then release it back into the wild the following day.

When the local team arrived at my house for a meeting the next morning, they saw the chameleon in the bucket, freaked out and walked right back out the door.

I followed them. 'What's the problem?'

'You cannot have chameleons in the house! This is very bad luck. We move out of houses when chameleons come in.'

I put the chameleon out in the backyard and promised the team I would set it free on my next trip to Zwedru, and they reluctantly agreed to come back inside and start the meeting. Later, I had trouble convincing my driver to take me to Zwedru with a chameleon in the car. He wouldn't leave unless the lizard rode in the boot in a sealed Tupperware container and made it about 600 metres up the road before insisting I set the thing free. *Alright, lesson learned regarding chameleons*, I thought.

A couple of days later, I had some visitors. There were two boys standing very proudly on my veranda with something that looked like a metal ball. My security guard explained that the boys had brought it for me because I had asked for it.

'Pardon?' I replied.

'They said you asked for this,' the guard repeated.

One of the boys gave the ball a shake and, *thwack*, out came a pangolin.

'Holy shit!' I exclaimed. It was like a Pokemon.

'We heard you like to buy these things,' said the boys.

'What? No!' I told them. 'Definitely not.'

I had never seen a pangolin before and it was utterly amazing.

'We're going to eat it if you don't buy it,' they said.

*Dammit.*

'No, I don't buy stuff. But I'll take a photo of it.'

I took a few snaps, feeling very sad for the poor pangolin, but knowing I had to draw the line before things got any worse. Of course, things got worse anyway. A few days later, my guard came in to let me know I had visitors again. I walked outside to find three guys sitting on a log with a baby chimpanzee on one of their laps.

*You are fucking kidding me*, I thought.

'We heard you to like to buy animals,' they said. I made one mistake with a chameleon and now in addition to going to environmental hell, WWF was going to throw me in jail. 'Do you want the monkey?' they asked.

'No, I don't want the monkey.'

'Then we will eat the monkey.'

'You're not going to eat the monkey!'

'We already ate the mother, we just thought you would like the baby.'

The chimpanzee reached out to me with its tiny little arms and jumped up into mine. I was on the verge of tears. 'You can't eat it!' I said quickly. 'Chimpanzees are full of disease. You could get sick. You never know what germs they have, these monkeys.'

Reluctantly, I let the little guy crawl back into their arms, hoping that I had bamboozled them with my hygiene talk. There was nothing else I could do. If I paid for the chimpanzee, they would only bring more, so I took a photo of the little thing and sent them on their way. But I made sure those guys told everyone in the village that I really, really, really didn't like animals.

We had cleared 600 metres of land when we found the tree. I don't know how we hadn't seen it previously—it was a towering giant with enormous roots that snaked over the ground—but it was impossible to miss once the jungle around it was gone. At its base, the tree must have been five or six metres in diameter. Its long trunk was completely bare until right up towards the top, where heavy branches sprouted into the sky. It was beautiful.

We decided to redesign the camp to create a child-friendly area in the shade of this mighty tree, with space allocated for traders around the edge of the clearing. I thought the community would really benefit from the adjustment, so I was very proud to tell Kate about it the next time she came down to visit.

'Look at this amazing tree!' I told her proudly. 'We're going to lose about ten tents, but we'll make it up elsewhere.'

When Kate went back to Zwedru she mentioned our tree in her cluster meeting and the next day two LandCruisers filled with officials came down to Ziah, including representatives from the forestry department. They took one look at it and told me, 'You cannot keep the tree.'

'What? Why?' I asked.

'This is a middle forest tree.'

'And?'

'And it is not in the middle of the forest anymore.'

The government officials explained that our tree was now far too exposed to the elements and would very likely fall down in a strong wind, which would be catastrophic. It was really massive. The officials couldn't help us remove the tree, but they insisted it had to go.

My de-foresting team took a good look at the trunk and said, 'We're going to need bigger chainsaws.'

We went over the plan hundreds of times. They would cut this way and then this way and then the tree would fall that way. We took down all the tents in a 300-metre radius just to be on the safe side, but the chainsaw team seemed confident that the tree would go in the right direction.

On the day of the big chop, I was called up to Zwedru and I felt very nervous about leaving the team alone, but what did I really know about cutting down trees? Not much. Anyway, the plan had been checked and re-checked, then checked again. The community had been prepared, there was a roped-off safety area policed by a team with radio communications, and we were as ready as we could be. I was due to be back by early afternoon and expected to see our mighty giant lying on the jungle floor.

When I got back, the tree was still there, upright. I called the team leader to figure out what had gone wrong. 'We've cut it down,' he told me, 'but it will not fall over.'

'What do you mean?'

He led me to the base of the trunk and showed me where they had cut, clean through to the other side. He had two of his team members pull a length of rope right through the cut, dragging it in between the stump and the trunk, while the trunk remained stubbornly vertical. 'It will not fall over,' the team leader shrugged.

The team had begun to chop into the trunk at angles, trying to destabilise it. They seemed confident that they would get it down eventually, so I left them to it and went for a tour of the community to make sure everyone was alright. When I came back a good hour later, the tree was still standing and people were starting to get nervous. The light was beginning to fade and it was getting close to dinnertime, so the community was moving around a little more, preparing food. It wasn't safe to leave things as they were.

We called a community meeting to form a new action plan. The people whose tents had been taken down had to be re-housed elsewhere for the night and we would need to pay people to stand guard over the tree and patrol the safety zone to keep people out. Afterwards, I radioed the chainsaw team to tell them to down tools. They couldn't hear me over the roar of the motor, so I walked into the safety zone to talk to the team leader. I walked in a straight line from the safety perimeter towards the crew, right in between two massive roots that were protruding from the ground.

I opened my mouth to say *You're going to have to stop*, but the words never came out. As I opened my mouth, the chainsaw team started running towards me. Without a sound, the massive fucking tree was falling.

Trapped between two roots, I could only run in one direction. Everything slowed down and I could hear my own heartbeat, thinking, *don't fall over, don't fall over, don't fall over.* Naturally, I fell over. In fact, I tripped into a hole. As I tried to pull myself up off the ground, I glanced up and saw a member of the chainsaw team; he was bare-chested, covered in sawdust, wearing my mirrored Oakley sunglasses. I had lent the sunglasses to him earlier because the sawdust was bothering his eyes. In slow motion, I saw the man spin around and run back towards me, then come to a skidding halt as he gazed upwards in horror. *Fuck, I'm fucked,* I thought. Then it was over.

I was choking on a cloud of dust, but I checked all my limbs and they were still there. I was lying in the dirt with the mammoth tree trunk lying right beside me where it had fallen, directly in between me and the community, which had taken a collective breath of fear. The last they had seen was me lying on the ground and the tree coming down in my general direction. Now that the tree was lying between us, they couldn't see anything at all.

When I stood up, my view was obscured by the tree's crumpled branches, so it took me a while to see anyone on the other side, until I spotted one of my drivers. He was on his knees with his head in his hands. I waved to signal to him and the whole crowd caught sight of me, and cheered like they had just won the World Cup.

'I'm okay!' I smiled, looking around to check if everyone else was also okay. I realised I had been cut rather badly so there was quite a bit of blood running down my arm, but I had already switched into command mode. 'Is everyone okay? Check every name. We need to get the tents back up before dark ...' As I spoke, the community swarmed around me, shouting joyfully and slapping me on the back and I felt quite overwhelmed for a second. *Fuck, that was close,* I thought. *That was really close.* But now there was work to do.

Later that night, I thought about it again. I sat alone in my house with no one to talk to, not even a drop of whisky to calm my nerves or celebrate my near miss. My arm needed stitches but I didn't have a kit, so I gave it a good clean and then sealed the wound with superglue, which worked just as well. When I was done, there was a knock at the door (finally, I had a door) and I walked outside to see about three hundred people from the refugee community sitting in my front yard. They said they were worried about me, but I assured them I was fine and that I'd see them in the morning. I waved them goodnight. I thought they went home but couldn't be sure, because they were sitting exactly where I left them when I emerged the next morning. Except now, at the front of the crowd, there were a bunch of people holding chickens.

The community was very spiritual and they believed that I had been cursed by something called the country devil, which was now determined to kill me. The community had kept a vigil outside my house to protect me overnight and they wanted to perform a ritual cleansing, which involved plucking feathers from the chickens and putting the feathers in my hair. *Oh Jesus*. I couldn't say no. These people, who days earlier had been eating jungle rats, had somehow managed to find a cluster of white chickens for the occasion and they were insisting I should take them.

'I can't take them!' I told the crowd.

'You cannot not take them,' they insisted. It was country devil business.

One by one, the people with chickens came up to me, plucked a ceremonial feather—*bwaaark!*—and put it in my hair, then handed me the chicken. I took the chickens, said thank you, and passed them to Angela. I was going to have to have some sort of roast chicken party. Later that same day, the chainsaw team arrived with a goat, because their bigger responsibility for the tree incident demanded a bigger sacrifice. *What part of that goes in my hair?* I wondered.

The final ritual came the following night. A group of men from Ziah set up a drumming circle at either end of my street and beat their drums nonstop until dawn. The next morning, they came to let me know that everything was fine. The country devil was gone for good. A few weeks later, with the camp nearly finished, my mission ended and I was gone, too.

# 17

# FAMINE, IN A BURKA AND RAY-BANS

I was exhausted after Liberia and I did nothing but sleep for several weeks. It became clear that my life in the field was catching up with me. It wasn't just the brucellosis or the whooping cough or the dengue fever or that last spectacular bout of gastro, it was the actual work. Roughing it out in remote areas, working intense schedules to get shit done—it was my absolute favourite thing in the world, but it was slowly killing me. My weight fluctuated wildly every time I went on a mission and I ended up in hospital more often than not. I joked about it but knew they were serious conditions that could have serious long-term effects. I was starting to feel really burnt out. My head and my heart wanted to keep going, but my body just needed to slow down.

I worked out a deal with Richard at Concern to ride a desk for a while, doing a little backline support for other people in the field. In 2012, there was a major drought and food insecurity crisis brewing in the Horn of Africa, and Concern had teams managing the problem in both Somalia and Kenya. Richard suggested I head to Kenya and work out of the office there.

Somalia was never an option. The team working there was entirely local because the security situation was far too volatile for expats—keeping us safe was just too much of a burden. But there was good internet service in Mogadishu and functional phone lines, so we provided remote support from Kenya and the local team ran the show.

My job was to check reports and proposals, provide secondary analysis and give advice by phone to the teams in Somalia and Kenya. I was based in Nairobi, a sprawling metropolis, the hub of major aid efforts by all the big organisations, including UNICEF and the World Food Programme, and of course the Red Cross. It was a collegial atmosphere and I found I quite liked it. I enjoyed being part of a team. The pace was also perfect—nine-to-five. In fact, technically, we finished at 4.30 p.m. because if we left any later it took two hours to get home. The traffic congestion in Nairobi made Kampala look like a country fair.

Getting posted to a major city meant living in relative luxury. I rented a really nice apartment—nice by my standards, anyway. It had windows, doors, running water and a bed, and a decent view over the city. I even had my own kitchenette, which meant I could start eating well. For the first time in years, I lived without a housekeeper, cook or cleaner. I had to pick up after myself and do my own shopping, just like a normal person. We often went out to dinner at one of Nairobi's many restaurants and on weekends we went shopping at the big mall in town, Westgate. It was the same place where sixty-seven people were killed by terrorists a few years later.

A— was now working in Geneva and we were in a long-distance relationship. Every romance I had had for nine years was long-distance, so it didn't seem unusual to me, but I was grateful to have a normal internet and phone service in Nairobi so that

I could speak to my partner every day. No more driving for two hours to the top of a hill in the hopes of getting a signal, no more bad connections or brief conversations because it was all too hard in the field.

I only left the office twice in Kenya. The Concern nutritionist took me out to see a program operating in Kibera, the largest urban slum in Africa, and later I went north to a town called Marsabit to see the drought firsthand. Marsabit looked like the moon, a baked seabed covered in rocks no bigger than your fist. I had never seen anything like it in my life; every last drop of moisture had been scorched away. Every drought scenario I had seen had been followed by a flood. I had never seen so many malnourished children in one spot, either. It wasn't just a lack of food; the kids were dying of thirst. Part of the Concern response involved trucking in water.

Despite all of this, the mayor of Marsabit was somehow convinced that the town was a tourist hot spot and he invited us to visit the national park nearby before we left the region. The park was just as dry as everywhere else—it looked like the whole thing would go up in flames if you threw a cigarette butt out of the window—and there was nothing to see, not even birds.

After a couple of hours of fruitless driving, we came to a lookout at the top of a hill and saw a vast meteorite crater on the plain below us. There was a pool of water in the very middle of the crater which had probably been a lake, but it had evaporated so much in the drought that it was now the size of a backyard swimming pool. Around the pool, there were more than a dozen elephants fighting for the last drop of water. *Jesus, we need a nutrition program for the elephants,* I thought. Even from our vantage point a kilometre away, we could see their rib cages protruding through their skin.

After the 1986 famine in Ethiopia, a number of early warning systems were put in place. There was a famine early warning system called FEWSNET which constantly tracked a number of indicators around household food security to make predictions around when issues would arise. The FEWSNET classification system included five phases: Minimal, Stressed, Crisis, Emergency and Famine. Famine was defined as 'an extreme lack of food and other basic needs where starvation, death, and destitution are evident'. It became a technical definition, tested against strict criteria and measurements. Since the FEWSNET system had been put into place, a famine had never been declared. Now, we were told a famine was coming in Somalia—a clear, unequivocal phase 5.

The problem was that the epicentre of the emergency was in southern Somalia, in a region called Shebelle, which was al-Shabaab territory. The Salafist jihadist military group controlled virtually everything south of Mogadishu and they had ejected most of the foreign aid organisations that were trying to deal with the crisis. Neither the UN's World Food Programme nor the Red Cross were welcome in al-Shabaab areas, so they had no access to the areas that were most affected by the drought.

Concern was still able to operate in Somalia because the local organisation had worked hard to develop relationships with the people in power, through an excellent country director who I will call Ibraahin. He ran a core team of Somali people who were able to negotiate with al-Shabaab to get access and run nutrition programs in the far south, but it was a very difficult landscape to operate in. Food and supplies were heavily taxed by the terrorist militia in the territories that most needed help.

All of the Horn of Africa was in a food security crisis, but the additional pressure applied by al-Shabaab is what triggered the famine in Shebelle. The political situation had overwhelmed the community's natural coping strategies to the point where people were starving to death. We were getting reports that people were trying to eat grass, or the straw roofs of their houses. Others became famine refugees, fleeing north towards Mogadishu, though al-Shabaab did their best to keep people trapped and under their control.

In total, 260,000 people would die in the Somali famine in just under five months.

The malnutrition program in Somalia had the same elements as the programs I had worked on previously—MUAC tape, Plumpy'Nut and supplementary food—but the whole famine response operated on a much broader scale. There were large-scale cash distribution and water-trucking projects, plus emergency housing and camp development projects responding to the mass migration of famine refugees. The population movement from Shebelle into lower Mogadishu was increasing daily, with almost a million people displaced over the course of the emergency.

I supported the malnutrition program remotely, giving advice and assistance to the teams in Somalia that were distributing Plumpy'Nut. The data I looked at every day was only one piece of the puzzle, but it very quickly illustrated the scale of the problem. I went to Kenya knowing that the situation would escalate but not prepared for how bad things would get.

Reports began to come in that there was a measles outbreak in Somalia, and measles and malnutrition don't go very well together. Measles was horrific anyway, but the first thing that happens to a child with measles is that they lose weight. The fatality rate for malnourished kids with measles was extremely high. I began to crunch the numbers, looking at the measles data alongside the global acute malnutrition rate. The GAM rate in

Somalia was 50 per cent—it had been 14 per cent in Niger—and half of the kids in Somalia qualified as severely malnourished. We were looking at a measles outbreak where roughly 50 per cent of infected children would die.

We then received word that there was a cholera outbreak in the refugee camps in Mogadishu. Cholera caused rice water diarrhoea so severe that patients were slung in hospitals beds with holes in them to allow the free flow of stool into a bucket beneath. With treatment, only 1 per cent of victims died from cholera. With no treatment, the fatality rate rose to 5 per cent. But when kids were malnourished and dehydrated, they really had no chance.

It was like one of those disaster movies: just when you thought it couldn't get any worse, it did. At the main public hospital, over half of the children in the malnutrition ward were dying within twenty-four hours of arrival. There was a clinic run by a small Turkish aid organisation where things were equally grim, and MSF reported that its malnutrition stabilisation centre was completely overwhelmed. Our own team reported that the Plumpy'Nut distribution program was straining under the load as well.

In Kenya, I started to write training programs to help our Somali team with the disease response. *What is measles? How do you care for a measles patient? How do you vaccinate?* They were basic, step-by-step guides to break down quite high-level technical information, written in the most foolproof language I could muster. I was on Skype with the local team every day to reinforce the lessons, walking them through all the instructions again via video link. It wasn't perfect, but it seemed like the only option.

Eventually, UNICEF approached Concern to ask for more assistance. Its own staff couldn't fly into Somalia, but the organisations that were operating in-country clearly needed some support. It seemed obvious that the Somali health teams were struggling to follow protocols, but we needed eyes on the ground. Someone needed to go in and provide training to bolster the emergency response. We discussed it and agreed that that someone was me.

Al-Shabaab was at Kilometre Six. The UN controlled the airport and a 6-kilometre stretch of territory from the airport into Mogadishu, but from Kilometre Six onwards the terrorist army had effective control. That 'safe zone' wasn't even the full radius of a circle, because the airport was built right on the coast.

Once Concern made the decision to send me, things moved very quickly because we didn't want to give people too much notice that I was on the way. We circulated a message to key aid organisations in-country: I would land in Somalia in two days for a week-long assessment and training program, and anyone working who wanted to was welcome to attend. We wanted to have as much impact as possible, and I was one of the few resources available.

Before I left Nairobi, I had to buy a burka. Somalia was a strict Islamic country, so I had to be covered at all times in the traditional religious dress. My hair had to be completely covered, my arms down to my wrists, and the burka had to fall all the way past my shoes to the floor. I tried to buy one at the market in Kenya, but I couldn't find anything off-the-shelf that reached further than my calves. In the end, one of the young Muslim women in our team took me burka shopping in the Indian quarter, where I could get one custom made. She tried to entice me with pink and blue fabrics. 'Black will do just fine,' I said. I looked pretty special when I boarded the plane—covered head-to-toe, wearing my Ray-Bans.

There was only one airline that flew into Somalia and it didn't inspire confidence. The armrests of my seat on the plane were held together with duct tape, and Mogadishu Airport wasn't in much better condition. The building looked similar to many others

I had been in in Africa, but there were no departure or arrival signs, no announcements, no crowd control. People seemed to move out onto the tarmac by instinct, just guessing when their plane was about to take off.

I went through a fairly loose customs process, filling out the necessary forms. The third question on my customs declaration form asked, 'What guns do you have and how much ammunition?' Not, *Are you carrying a weapon?* Just, *Which ones do you have?*

Ibraahin, the Concern country director, was waiting for me in the arrival hall. He led me out of the building and beyond the first safety perimeter to where three Concern vehicles were waiting for us. In the middle, with completely blacked-out windows, was a Toyota Hilux four-wheel drive. On either side, there were tray-back trucks carrying what we called 'technical teams'. In the tray of each truck, a guy stood beside a 50-millimetre machine gun. Surrounding them, in the tray and the cab of the vehicles, were several other men carrying heavy weapons and ammunition.

I was ushered into the middle car with Ibraahin, and seated behind yet another guy with a huge gun. With the technical teams as our escort, we drove 4 kilometres to the Concern compound in Mogadishu. I have no idea where it was. They took backstreets, at speed, going out of their way repeatedly, so that a 4-kilometre trip took the better part of fifteen minutes. It was standard protocol for losing potential attackers.

As we drove, the streets of Mogadishu slipped by, a surprisingly beautiful city. The Arjuran Sultanate had left a stunning archaeological legacy, with ruined castles and fortresses dotted along the coast. The Italian occupation in the early twentieth century had created a ton of impressive architecture as well, including the Mogadishu Cathedral, which rose up beside the Arba'a Rukun Mosque.

I glimpsed all of this through the window, through a teeming sea of bodies. Mogadishu was completely overrun with internally displaced people. Shelters were thrown up on every footpath, made from pieces of tarpaulin or empty hessian bags which had once held food rations distributed by the UN. Every inch of space was occupied with makeshift refugee camps.

The security teams were hyper vigilant. There was constant radio chatter as we drove and they moved quickly into position when we arrived at the Concern compound. The car in front of us moved to block the street while the massive compound gate rolled open. We swung into the compound without stopping, the other cars close behind us. The guards jumped out immediately, checking the sky and the perimeter walls—a confident and well-oiled machine.

Concern rarely worked with guns but there was plenty of security expertise within the team and they had operated in Somalia throughout the civil war, including the period described in the film *Black Hawk Down*. Ibraahin was very well connected, very experienced and set high safety standards. He told me that I couldn't stay at the Concern compound for long. I would meet briefly with the team and then I would be taken back to a secure hotel within the Kilometre Four safe zone.

Back at the hotel, I met with Ibraahin for a full security briefing. Sitting on plastic chairs on the hotel terrace, I could hear the Indian Ocean, but there was a three-metre wall between me and the view, patrolled by armed guards. Ibraahin introduced me to the head of the security team, who told me to think of myself as a walking ATM. He was blunt and no-bullshit. I was a million dollars on legs, he said, which meant that I would be safe. When I got kidnapped I shouldn't worry because I was too valuable to kill and it was only a matter of time before Concern negotiated my release. He said 'when', not 'if'.

This wasn't the situation everywhere in the world. If an aid worker was captured in Afghanistan or Pakistan, there was every chance they would be beheaded in a terrorist propaganda video, but kidnapping in Somalia was a livelihood activity. I would likely be held for twelve to eighteen months, but eventually released. The key to surviving was to stay focused and motivated. I figured I could run a little primary school or clinic to pass the time. I would exercise, lose some weight, and come out looking like Linda Hamilton in *Terminator 2*. I had a whole plan worked out in my head.

The security guy told me that my kidnappers would charge Concern fifty dollars a day while I was held, but this would ensure I had enough food and water. He introduced me to a man who would be my 'chef' while I was in captivity and asked me to come up with a code word we could share in order to communicate safely. I suggested 'wombat', which was a hangover from Aceh. The expat team in Indonesia had dared me to drop strange words randomly into a media interview and 'wombat' was the only word I had never managed to sneak in. Unfortunately, the chef had no idea what a wombat was so there was no chance he would remember it. We decided my code word in Somalia would be 'strawberries'.

The head of security stressed that I shouldn't worry too much about being kidnapped, but it was important that I understood the threat. There were no more than fifteen expats in Mogadishu at one time, so if a kidnapping did happen, the odds of it being me were roughly one in fifteen. The more people in town, the lower the risk. If the security team learned that other foreigners had flown out, then I would be flying out, too. Too few expats in town meant too much risk.

I was warned to wear sturdy and comfortable clothing at all times, because whatever I was wearing on the day I was kidnapped would be the clothes I wore for the next twelve to eighteen months. But it was so unbelievably hot, I ended up dressing for the weather. Under my burka, I wore Blundstones, a pair of Billabong shorts and a Chesty Bonds singlet, although I always made sure I was wearing a sturdy bra. *If only they knew I was wearing fewer clothes than usual under this thing.*

The whole time I was in Somalia, I never felt uneasy. The security team was so professional and alert that I felt very well protected. Not being responsible for my own security had a lot to do with it. My safety was in the hands of people whose primary job was to keep me safe. There were a lot of rules, and all I had to do was follow them. I was cool with that. And whatever the risk, given the crisis we were facing, I felt like it was worth it.

Alongside the local Concern team, my first training program in Somalia included nursing teams from the main public hospital, the Turkish hospital and a small aid organisation called SOS, which ran a training clinic in Mogadishu. It lasted a week. I wore my burka all day, every day, but I never quite got the knack of it. The headscarf was a tricky piece of material and it was constantly slipping off my head. Eventually the local team took pity on me and bought me a training hijab with elastic around the face, meant for little girls. Made all the difference.

What became apparent very quickly was that no one knew the correct protocols for treating malnourished kids. The Turkish team had been feeding the kids with milk and figs, and putting IV drips in to rehydrate them quickly. The kids had a high fatality rate, but the team had no idea why: the chemistry of the kids' bodies was so out of whack that the diet was probably causing cardiac overload. It's not that they were killing the kids, but their patients weren't recovering from the malnutrition and they were getting worse rapidly. In the main hospital, the staff was giving the kids IV drips but they weren't feeding them regularly. They were also keeping measles patients and malnourished patients in the same ward.

These were fairly clear problems with simple solutions. We focused on basic clinical protocols: *this is how you diagnose; this is how often you feed; this is how you prevent cross-contamination.* The Turkish team had never heard of Plumpy'Nut, so we were able to completely overhaul their program by supplying them with the right products and medications. Within weeks, their fatality rate dropped dramatically and they were training people outside their own team.

The fatality rate for the malnourished kids in the main hospital was 25 per cent when I arrived—vastly higher than acceptable standards. We worked on the hospital's hygiene, nutrition and safe hydration standards, and as a result the case fatality rate also dropped rapidly, down to 11 per cent. This happened just a week after I'd left Mogadishu. People had applied the training and the impact was immediate.

When I landed back in Kenya, Ibraahin called to let me know that the feedback had been incredible. The head of the main public hospital was implementing major changes and people were responding very proactively across the board, but there were still significant gaps in knowledge in the local teams. The gaps extended beyond the nutrition and health programming, too; the massive influx of refugees into Mogadishu had created significant water and sanitation challenges in the camps. Ibraahin and I had discussed these issues before I left the country and I'd made some recommendations that were useful. He wondered if there was more I could contribute.

'Would you be willing to come back and run some training sessions on water and sanitation?' he asked. *What else could you do?*

*What else could you teach us?* There was an incredible hunger within the local teams to learn and improve their service delivery. They were determined not to be overwhelmed by the crisis.

Over the next nine weeks, I flew into Mogadishu half a dozen times to deliver more training. I ran programs on cholera, measles, nutrition, water and sanitation and refugee camp management; dehydration, rehydration; hygiene promotion and water chlorination. Sometimes I was there for a week at a stretch; other times I would only last a few days before I got the call from Ibraahin to say I was being evacuated. They kept an ear to the ground, responded to rumours quickly and moved me around rapidly.

I was very motivated, but it was a hammering experience. On every flight out of Mogadishu, I had to go through heavy security with a full body search, then halfway to Nairobi the plane would stop in the desert town of Wajir. Everyone had to disembark and all the luggage was taken off the plane, and we were subjected to another full security check while our bags went through an X-ray scan. We then reboarded and continued to Nairobi airport, only to be held in a secure room until all the luggage was checked again. We were then called from the room one by one and sent through to the regular immigration checkpoint. It took three hours to fly into Somalia, but eight or nine hours to get out. Once, I was sent a text message before I had even landed in Kenya to let me know I would be on a plane back to Somalia the following afternoon. Seemed funny to me that I had felt tired before.

Despite the fatigue, I enjoyed being able to socialise in Nairobi, taking full advantage of the access to proper food and good restaurants when I was back in the city. And besides, who knew how long I would have access to such amenities? Maybe my next trip would be the one when I was abducted. This was my justification for the overindulgence that resulted in what I jokingly called my 'emergency ration pack'—an extra 8 kilograms of soft belly. Unfortunately, I wasn't kidnapped, so I kept the emergency ration pack long after the mission ended.

When I was in Mogadishu, I was confined to the hotel or the Concern compound, where the nursing teams and doctors came to me for their training and technical support. Only twice was I allowed to go anywhere else: once to a camp for internally displaced people and once to a nutrition centre in the middle of the city. In both instances, I was only allowed out of the vehicle for twenty minutes. We arrived in a convoy with the technical teams and I had twenty minutes to jump out and do a visual assessment before the guards whisked me back into the car and back to the Concern compound. They knew that word would get out that I was on site, but it would take a would-be attacker at least twenty minutes to mobilise and get to our location. We would be gone by then.

The nutrition centre was a small corrugated shed on the side of a road, completely surrounded by an informal refugee camp. People had set up whatever they could, however they could, throwing up tarpaulins and tents on every spare centimetre of ground. Inside, the nutrition centre looked much like the ones I had seen else-where. The mothers were lined up around the edge of the building with their children in their laps; the kids were eating Plumpy'Nut in preparation for their appetite test. There were children being weighed and assessed, and boxes of Plumpy'Nut being handed out. The only major problem they had at the centre was how to manage the volume of people who were coming in every day.

We did a quick assessment of how the kids were flowing through the program and where bottlenecks were occurring, and found that things were piling up around the weighing station. It was taking the mothers too long to get their kids undressed, so I suggested getting the mothers to undress their children while they were waiting. The Concern team was using little pants that acted as a harness for the weighing process, but they presented an infection risk for measles and cholera, so I suggested they change to a bucket weighing system that could be cleaned quickly. I realised there was no triage process for kids who were sick, so we established that at the entry point. The Plumpy'Nut distribution was also very slow, but they could improve the process by pre-packing kits according to the children's weight range. In twenty minutes, we identified a host of small solutions that together would make a big difference.

I really wanted to visit the public hospital. The fatality rate there had dropped, but the doctors were still calling me with various issues and I really needed to be able to see what they were seeing. The difficulty was that a number of improvised explosive devices (IEDs) had been detonated near the hospital because that was where journalists had gathered to report on the famine. It was stressful enough for the technical teams when I was at lower-risk sites, so visiting the hospital was really out of the question. I would just have to get creative.

I asked the team to go to the market and buy me a video camera, and we hired a cameraman to go to the hospital each day and film everything that was going on. I would sit with him in the morning and give him an observational checklist, and in the evening I would sit down with the various health teams and go through the footage. For the most part, the conditions were as expected. Overcrowding, no running water, no support services. There were also some very obvious hygiene issues, like no waste bins. The mothers were throwing dirty nappies out of the windows and you could see them hanging in the trees outside the hospital. There were no handwashing stations, either, and very little in terms of general upkeep. These things, at least, were relatively easy to fix. Concern was able to buy bins and materials for handwashing stations, and hire cleaners to improve the overall hygiene conditions. With these changes, we were able to bring the child fatality rate down by a few more points.

Being a paediatric nurse, working in a measles and cholera outbreak in the middle of a famine, teaching and developing skills, and seeing a real and measurable impact—all of this was incredibly motivating. It required the cumulative experience of my entire professional life; it was like the public health Olympics, and I was in the decathlon. Of all the big, dramatic results I had thrived on during my career, these made me the most proud. So while the famine was devastating and the casualties were enormous, Somalia was actually a very positive experience for me.

The most amazing element of all of this was the local teams. I had never seen such dedication and tenacity, coupled with such joyful enthusiasm for the work. These guys operated in incredibly dangerous and challenging conditions, but they never complained. They jumped at any chance they had to make things better, however small. They wanted to learn and they wanted to help people, and they were grateful that they had the opportunity to do that. They were incredibly inspiring.

But there were other people who were affected by this mission who weren't having such a great time. Not only did my trips into Mogadishu cause huge stress for the local security teams, but my friends and family at home were more worried about me than they had ever been. Having a partner in the field wasn't fun for A——, who probably worried the most.

There were always gunshots being fired in Mogadishu, but they were usually far away, or the recognisable pattern of my guards clearing their weapons. I only tuned in when the burst of sound was somehow unfamiliar. I was skyping A— one day when a few volleys rang out very close to the hotel, so I climbed under the desk as I had been trained to do.

'What are you doing?' A— asked. 'Is that gunfire?'

'Oh, it's probably just the security guards,' I lied, now sitting on the floor.

Outside, the rapid exchange of rounds continued, but I never found out what it was.

Later, an expat working for MSF was killed at the compound just across from mine. He had sacked a member of his local staff, who had returned later to execute him and the head of his local team. I was 40 metres away when it happened, but this time I didn't hear a thing.

I wasn't afraid. I didn't expect anything to happen to me, but I was constantly alert and aware of my surroundings, and that was an insidious form of stress. It was a quiet, grinding physical strain on top of the pressures of the work, and I had to admit that it was starting to affect my health. Kenya was supposed to be downtime but I had managed to drag myself into Somalia and, unexpectedly, that had taken me to the end of the line.

Over the years I had seen more than one humanitarian aid worker become a cautionary tale, burned out after years of hard living with no roots and no boundaries, their bodies taxed and their family lives a train wreck. I had made a pact with some colleagues in Aceh to make sure I never ended up that way. When I got the job with Concern, I spoke to my friends and warned them that I would probably like the work too much and would need someone to tell me when it was time to leave. That time had snuck up on me.

I came home from Somalia with antibiotic-resistant conjunctivitis, impetigo and a mouth full of ulcers.

A— said, 'That's enough, you need to stop.'

# 18

## Saving the World, one Email at a Time

There was always a bit of tension between people in the field and people at headquarters. Concern was actually pretty good at listening to the 'voice from the field', but in the humanitarian industry generally, there was often a disconnect between the high-level planning and strategy, and the realities on the ground. I never wanted to be a 'headquarters' person, but the time had come. I needed to give my body a break and my relationship a proper go. Living out of a suitcase wasn't good for me; I needed to put down some roots. This suited A— just fine.

It meant that I would need to look for a job in Geneva—the humanitarian capital of the world—but it had to be the right job. I loved working for Concern and I didn't really want to leave, but I figured it would take a few months at least to find something interesting, so I would have time to ease into the idea. As it happened, I found something interesting about a week in: an advertisement for the Global Emergency Health Advisor with the International Federation of the Red Cross, the largest humanitarian organisation in the world. The role described was the perfect balance of technical advice and field support—the best of both worlds.

I expected a lengthy vetting and interview process. I had had three interviews and an exam before I joined Concern, and the Federation job seemed a much higher level to me, so I expected to jump through a few hoops before I knew what was happening. I didn't think to let Richard at Concern know that I had applied.

Shortly after I sent in my résumé, I was in Rome to deliver a conference paper on the Concern mission in Uganda when I got a call to say that the Federation wanted to interview me. Over Skype, they asked four or five fairly easy questions. I actually thought I had blown the interview and they'd stopped before they got to the tricky ones, but the next morning when I woke up, they had emailed me an offer. They wanted me to be in Geneva within a couple of weeks to get started.

Leaving Concern was like breaking up with someone. I flew to Dublin and sat down with Richard over a cup of Earl Grey tea and told him, 'It's not you, it's me.' He completely understood that I needed a more stable life and said, 'We can make it work!' We discussed some possible scenarios where I worked out of Geneva for Concern, but ultimately it was just too hard. Heartbreaking, but too hard. I was headed back to the Red Cross.

A— had already been living in Geneva for six months and was all set up in a cosy one-bedroom apartment. Rent was exorbitant, particularly for such a small place. The studio would do for the time being, but you couldn't swing a cat. I hadn't paid rent since I lived in Alice Springs; literally every home I'd had when I was working had been provided as part of the job. I had hardly cleaned my own house in over eight years. I hardly even drove a car anymore. Now I was going to set up house, with a domestic partner and domestic responsibilities. There were moments of pure panic.

I had to buy new clothes. My uniform of jeans, Blundstone boots and polo shirts had served me well for years, but was not going to cut it at Federation headquarters. I was a working stiff now. On my first day of work, A— surprised me with a gift: a coffee cup, a photo frame and a ceramic scuba diving cow to put on my desk. Apparently people liked personnel knick-knacks to personalise their office space. Who knew?

I caught public transport to the Federation 'house' every morning and sat in what seemed to be an endless procession of meetings, and when I wasn't doing that, I answered emails all day long. It wasn't my natural environment and I struggled at first. The work was interesting, it was actually quite important, but it was an adjustment. I was saving the world one email at a time.

When I first started, I was responsible for providing technical support to all Red Cross health operations in Africa and the Asia-Pacific—a huge chunk of the globe to cover. In any one day, I could be providing support on multiple diseases or operations, from an earthquake in Asia to multiple disease outbreaks at different scales within Africa. Zika, yellow fever, cyclones, malaria, floods, malnutrition—it all crossed my desk.

Years of study had given me a strong theoretical and technical knowledge covering a wide variety of disasters and emergencies, but being able to put my field lens over things definitely helped. I had a good understanding of what was practical and doable in most emergency scenarios. If a team in the field called to say that they couldn't move equipment because a road had disappeared, or that the ministry of health was blocking them, or that a community engagement strategy didn't seem to be working, I knew what they meant. I'd been there, so it was easy for me to help them find solutions.

The program design was very different to Concern's—large integrated programs like I had run in Niger were not really appropriate. The national Red Cross societies that were strong and robust didn't need our support. For the most part, I worked with the national societies that didn't have enough staff, or enough money, or enough technical knowledge. Their strength was that they had volunteers everywhere, all across any given country, which gave us a unique level of access into the community. The trick was to figure how to activate those volunteers in simple, effective ways.

This is assuming that the national societies were interested in my help. The running joke about my role was that while it was in my job description to provide technical support and advice, it wasn't in anyone's job description to accept it.

When people weren't coming to me for assistance, I was looking for trouble. Data mining was a big part of my job with the Federation, which meant scanning the internet to look for signs of coming health emergencies around the world. There were key sites like FEWSNET and another one called ProMED, which collated data about infectious disease and sent out regular updates, but a lot of my research involved scanning daily news bulletins. From the BBC and CNN, I'd harvest information about political instability in Africa and the Asia-Pacific, which was one of the biggest risk factors when it came to public health. If a natural disaster or major accident struck unexpectedly, I often saw it on the news first.

I had a global overview with information from lots of different sources and it was my role to analyse the risks and communicate them down the chain. If I came across any red flags, I would call the teams in the field and ask if anything was on their radar.

*I've heard there's some cholera here, have you followed up on it?* More often than not, my call was the first time the local team had heard about it. My job was to have eyes everywhere, to communicate with the people who could respond, and to make sure they had the resources they needed as quickly as possible.

The other significant part of my role with the Federation was the least familiar to me when I started out: global representation, leadership and advocacy for the Red Cross. I was now part of a cohort of international aid agencies, researchers and technicians that worked together on global strategies to respond to public health emergencies—a group of 200–300 people responsible for the big picture, including representatives from the UN, WHO and MSF.

It was very cool to meet with people who had extraordinarily high-level information about public health and disease, and still have something to contribute, though I sometimes sat in full-day meetings where I hardly understood anything anyone was saying. Some of the experts I sat with were so specialised they could talk for hours not just on one disease, but on one small characteristic of one disease. I once spent a whole day in a meeting about the shortage of sterile chicken eggs in Russia, which were needed as part of the process to produce yellow fever vaccine. No eggs, no vaccine, it seemed, but it took about eight hours to say that. That there were people who sat around all day worrying about chicken eggs was quite the revelation.

My role was to be a translator, bringing information from the field into these high-level meetings, explaining the complexities and difficulties of actually implementing programs, and then interpreting the science or recommendations from these meetings back down to the field teams in a way that could be translated into action.

*How am I going to explain this to the volunteers and how will they explain it to the community?*

*That's great, but the community would never accept it.*

*That's great, but we won't be able to implement the program in that way.*

*We're going to need to consider weather/culture/religious factors when rolling this out.*

I added a social mobilisation and community aspect to global strategy discussions, and gradually was asked to bring that viewpoint to public health conferences around the world. My message was always the same: *the community needs to be at the centre of all health emergency planning.* It's funny how often that commonsense advice came as a surprise.

I didn't plan to end up where I was. Every step in my career had felt very natural, and each mission and position had built on the one before, carrying me forward until I found myself with this really fascinating global overview. It happened by accident rather than by design, but every step I took along the way prepared me for what was to come.

What I liked most about my job with the Federation was that I still had a connection to the field. I bridged the space between the high-level management side of humanitarian aid and the coalface of program delivery, and it was a nice position to be in. I felt like a useful cog in the machine that made the humanitarian system run.

I deployed to the field occasionally to support different Red Cross operations, including a cholera response in Sierra Leone in 2012 and the Typhoon Haiyan response in 2013. My field kit stayed packed and ready to go, always. Some habits were hard to break, but I also believed that staff at headquarters needed regularl reality checks. Seeing how things were implemented on the ground allowed me to develop new tools and improve the guidance and advice I was doling out. It helped to understand where the bottlenecks were and what support we could provide to unblock the operations.

Besides, the Red Cross volunteers were like crack for me. They were the perfect antidote to the politics and the bureaucratic battles I came up against in Geneva. If I ever felt like I was losing perspective, the commitment and energy of the volunteers inspired me to work harder and do better. They believed in the Red Cross like it was a religion, and I believed in them.

# 19

# LOVE IN A TIME OF EBOLA

*UNDIAGNOSED VIRAL HAEMORRHAGIC FEVER - GUINEA:*
*EBOLA CONFIRMED*
★★★★★★★★★★★★★★★★★★★★★★★★★★★★★★★★★★★★★★★★★★★★★★★★★★★★★★★★

*A ProMED-mail post*
*http://www.promedmail.org*
*ProMED-mail is a program of the International Society for Infectious Diseases*
*http://www.isid.org*

*Date: Sat 22 Mar 2014*
*Source: BBC News*

*The Ebola virus has been identified as the cause of an outbreak of haemorrhagic fever now believed to have killed nearly 60 people in southern Guinea, government officials say.*

*Scores of cases have been recorded since the outbreak began early last month [February 2014].*

*There is no known cure or vaccine for the highly contagious Ebola virus. It is spread by close personal contact with people who are infected and kills between 25 percent and 90 per cent of victims.*

On 29 March 2014, ProMED put out an alert for an undiagnosed haemorrhagic fever in the West African country of Guinea. I was always on the lookout for outbreaks of haemorrhagic fever— a collection of virus symptoms including internal and external bleeding—because the range of diseases that produced these symptoms were highly infectious and often fatal. Any haemor-rhagic fever outbreak required a quick and careful response. In some instances, just one case was defined as an emergency.

The ProMED report caught my attention for personal reasons, too. A—'s doctoral work had focused on the exact same area of Guinea. My partner knew the area very well and had always wanted to study a haemorrhagic fever outbreak, so I knew A— would be excited about it. Sure enough, A— called me from the MSF offices in Geneva shortly after the alert came in. The organ-isation was mobilising an outbreak investigation team which would fly into Guinea the next day to start tracing the chain of transmission. A— wanted my blessing to go, because it was dangerous work. Who was I to stand in my partner's way?

On 22 March, the haemorrhagic fever was confirmed as the Ebola virus. Patient zero was a two-year-old boy named Emile who was thought to have contracted it from a dead bat in the Guinean forest, in the district of Guéckédou. He had passed the infection to his mother, sister and grandmother. Like Emile, they had died. Mourners at the grandmother's funeral then carried the virus to other villages in the region.

By the time WHO formally announced the outbreak on 23 March, more than eighty people were believed to be infected in Guinea, with at least sixty deaths. The following day, Liberia announced six suspected cases and five deaths. Ebola was on the move.

The IFRC deployed a medical team to Guinea on 24 March, led by my colleague Charles, while I stayed in Geneva to manage logistics and deployments. In the first few weeks of the emergency, I had an unusual level of insight for someone who wasn't in the field because A— was calling me two or three times a day from Guéckédou, where the outbreak was already out of control. MSF had set up an isolation and treatment centre but it was already full, so people were unable to access care and they were literally dying in the street.

From the ground, A— reported that there was no coordinated response system, not enough resources, only chaos. The IFRC volunteers in Guinea were especially vulnerable, A— said.

In health emergencies, the IFRC was responsible for social mobilisation, which meant talking to the community, letting everyone know about the disease, about what causes it and what symptoms to look out for. Ebola was particularly difficult because it had never been seen in that part of West Africa before. It ripped through the community so quickly, with symptoms so intense and terrifying, that a whole lot of misinformation began circulating, which only made things worse.

It was a politically fraught situation in Guinea because the local population was wary of its own political leadership, and the lack of trust in local authorities led to a lack of trust in the information that the community was receiving about Ebola. As the death toll climbed, so did the hysteria. Rumours began to circulate that the MSF team in Guéckédou was performing medical tests and harvesting organs in the isolation centre, because people who went in never came out. The fatality rate from Ebola was so high that it was true, most people who went in came out in body bags, but the confusion and fear around what was going on kept highly contagious patients out with the general population, infecting between two and twenty other people before they died. The IFRC teams were struggling to get people to understand why they had to be isolated, why they couldn't touch anyone and why they couldn't bury their dead in the normal way.

My job, in part, was to get the local IFRC team some materials to help manage the situation. A year earlier, I had deployed to a small Ebola outbreak in Uganda which had ended very quickly, and afterwards I sat with the IFRC volunteers and the community to discuss the messaging they had used during the outbreak. In Uganda, the campaign posters and flyers had read, 'Ebola kills. There is no cure.' These were messages carried not just by the national IFRC society, but by MSF and the Ugandan ministry of health. The IFRC doesn't usually use such negative language because it can create a stigma that does more harm than good, but a review showed that those fearmongering messages had driven community change very quickly in Uganda, which is one of the reasons the outbreak had been contained.

We sent the material from the Ugandan Ebola response to the IFRC society in Guinea to be translated into French and adapted for the local context, but the effect was very different. So little was known and understood about the disease in the community that such messaging didn't result in behaviour change, it only resulted in more fear. We heard rumours that entire villages had become infected, but had cut down trees to block the roads and prevent any assistance from reaching them. Once people had become that frightened, the stress impeded logic and even self-preservation instincts. This is one of the reasons that the epidemic raged out of control.

In those early weeks, we realised that mistakes had been made, that the messaging was wrong, and responded as quickly as we could. One of the earliest survivors in the MSF isolation clinic was recruited to work for the organisation, talking to the community about his experience. One of the things he was most positive about regarding the isolation centre was the endless supply of decent food and Coke, which was seen as a great enticement. MSF also took down the fence around the centre in Guéckédou so that people could see inside. It compromised patient dignity in some ways, but put an end to the fearmongering around organ harvesting. Families could now see in, and visit patients. We then started monitoring social media for unhelpful rumours circulating in the community, and did our best to shut them down before they did any damage. But things were moving so fast it was hard to keep up.

In Guinea, the infections had spread west along the main road from Guéckédou to Conakry on the coast. Our initial deployment of French doctors and nurses was spread along this route to support the local teams, but there were massive frustrations at every turn which impeded their work.

The local team members of the Guinea IFRC society team had no access to bank accounts, so we couldn't transfer funds to support them. They were overwhelmed—a highly committed but very small and under-resourced team—and their vehicles were barely roadworthy. MSF was desperate for extra staff and had begun training the local IFRC to deal with dead body management, then complained to us that the work wasn't being done. In their haste to recruit qualified people for their own operations, MSF had employed the three most senior staff members of the Guéckédou IFRC team, and without them, the network of volunteers had collapsed.

Meanwhile, the dead body management was incredibly fraught. Ebola was transmitted by contact with the body fluids of an infected person—blood, sweat, vomit, diarrhoea—and the virus load was at its peak when a person died. Dead bodies were highly infectious and needed to be handled with extreme caution and specific safety protocols, involving a team of four or five people in full Personal Protective Equipment (PPE)—yellow 'hazmat' coveralls with full face protection and gloves. The bodies were sprayed with a chlorine solution to inactivate the virus, then lifted into a heavy duty body bag. Early in the outbreak, they double-bagged the corpses so that nothing would leak out, then buried them. When this was done, the dead body management team had to remove their PPE, generally in uncontrolled environments, often outdoors, which was the highest point of risk to their own safety. It was especially challenging in an environment where the community didn't always understand or support the precautions.

Traditional burials in that part of Guinea involved washing the corpse, with the same water then used to cleanse the people who had performed the ritual. If the person had died from Ebola, that water was guaranteed to be infected, but the ritual had important religious meaning for the community. In a time of crisis, people clung to their faith.

We heard that a traditional healer had contracted Ebola in Guéckédou after treating dozens of patients, and hundreds of people had come to her funeral, carrying her body through the streets. Sixty or seventy people may have been contaminated as a result, some of whom had carried the disease across the border, into Sierra Leone.

Back in Geneva, I was fielding journalists and media interrogation at every turn. I went to a UN press conference in an attempt to explain what was happening: we were facing a major health emergency, the chain of transmission tracing was still not clear and that the outbreak was getting exponentially worse. As MSF had indicated, the geographic spread of the disease was already unprecedented and was out of control. A representative from WHO disagreed. He said that while he understood the concerns of MSF and the IFRC, this was a disease that did not normally result in a lot of cases. He was right, the largest outbreak previously had maxed out at about 600 cases, but this was clearly different. Ebola normally occurred in remote, isolated villages. This outbreak had already spread well beyond one village and was on the move.

Internally, at the Federation, we were also struggling to get support during those initial weeks. The Federation was a huge machine and worked best in large earthquakes and tsunamis. It was an amazing engine, really formidable when it kicked into gear, but Ebola needed a different style of response. The response needed to be dynamic and agile in order to move quicker than the disease. We had health teams in all three countries that were affected, but we needed additional support in terms of coordination, logistics and support services. The outbreak wasn't seen as big enough to warrant the deployment.

The Federation had responded to every Ebola outbreak since it was discovered in 1976, but it normally did so by releasing funds to the national IFRC and Red Crescent societies and providing a few key technical people for support. As the outbreak developed, the need for more international support was obvious. In the affected countries, the ministry of health teams were collapsing under the pressure while MSF was already under strain and stretched. They clearly needed our help, but when we raised a request for medical teams to deploy, no one responded. The national societies around the world were struggling to comprehend how bad the situation could get and we hadn't really prepared our medical teams for this type of work. The national societies were also concerned about deploying their teams in such an unstable landscape, when the protocols for managing the evacuation of infected IFRC and Red Crescent staff had yet to be nutted out.

Every day, we fought for more support, for more attention to be paid to the crisis, and worked with the teams on the ground to provide whatever assistance we could. I was deeply involved in the Ebola response, but all from the comfort of my desk in Geneva. And being that far away from the action was starting to drive me crazy. I had all this nervous energy that needed to be let out, so I started building. While A— was in Guinea, I built a 3.5 by 3-metre set of shelves in our apartment out of steel pipes and wood. We had no car, so I made multiple trips between the hardware store and our house on public transport, fielding phone calls about Ebola in either direction.

When A— came back from the field, a few months after deploying, we planned to take a couple of weeks off to go camping in Mongolia. On consideration, we decided it against it. A— was absolutely wrecked and I wasn't much better off, so we rented a villa with a pool in Malta instead and we both slept for the better part of a week.

The day after I got back, I got a call from my boss. We had reached the tipping point: the Director-General of WHO had called the Secretary General of the Federation to make a direct plea for support, and we had the green light to send in expat medical teams. I was being deployed to an Ebola mission in Sierra Leone.

I knew the IFRC society in Sierra Leone well because we had worked together during the 2012 cholera outbreak and I returned briefly in May 2014 for an evaluation of the response. My trip was before the first Ebola case was declared in Sierra Leone, but the local IFRC team was already deep into their preparedness strategy. The disaster management team had made T-shirts for the volunteers, and they were very proud to show me one when I visited. It had a massive skull and crossbones in the centre and read, 'Keep Ebola out of Sierra Leone!'

'So, guys, in terms of health promotion, what are we trying to say here?' I asked diplomatically. The pirate symbol was particularly disturbing. I asked how many they had printed—only two. *Good, let's keep it that way.*

Shortly afterwards, on 24 May, the first Ebola case was declared in Sierra Leone. By mid-June, there were more than a hundred cases in the country, rising rapidly. The WHO had six staff members working out of a hospital in the district of Kenema, but they were completely overwhelmed. I was deployed to set up an overflow ward, leading a construction and clinical team to bolster their capacity.

On my way to Kenema, I stopped in the Sierra Leone capital of Freetown and had a meeting with the IFRC society. One of the volunteers complained that he had been awake since two o'clock in the morning because he had been woken by a text message from his relative. In the middle of the night, a religious leader in Freetown had decreed that anyone who got up, washed in salt water and read a psalm from the Bible would be saved from Ebola, and the man had done as instructed.

'Oh really?' I replied in surprise.

According to the morning news bulletin, more than 1.5 million people had done it, the man said. I looked around the table. 'How many of you did it?' Every single hand went up. 'But why?!'

The secretary general of the Sierra Leone IFRC looked at me very evenly and said, 'Amanda, will washing in salt water hurt us?'

'No.'

'Will saying a prayer hurt us?'

'No.'

'Then we might as well give it a try.'

These people were my link to the community in Sierra Leone, but it was obvious that they too were consumed by fear.

The IFRC had never done clinical treatment of Ebola before. In previous outbreaks, MSF had always taken the lead and had managed to contain them, but this was more than MSF could handle on its own. It was already running four major treatment centres in three countries. The MSF doctors needed back-up, so they offered to train us, in the hope we could pick up some of the strain.

MSF had established a hundred-bed treatment unit in Kailahun, Sierra Leone, just south of the border from Guéckédou. It was the largest Ebola treatment centre that had ever been established, though it would soon be dwarfed by a 400-bed unit in Liberia. Kailahun was my first stop after Freetown. There, I was supposed to learn exactly how to build and operate an Ebola treatment centre. It's not like I had ever done it before.

The first thing the unit manager said to me was, 'I am really sorry, but I've got no time for you.'

'I understand, but if you guys want an overflow unit in Kenema, I'm going to need some guidance.'

'One of my logisticians can spend an hour with you tomorrow,' she said. That was the best I was going to get under the circumstances.

The next morning, the logistician showed me some basic schematic drawings of what an Ebola treatment centre should look like—the isolation ward, green 'safe' zones, decontamination points, a PPE removal zone—and then took me on a short tour of the facility. Chlorine was the main tool for decontamination and they were piping it pre-mixed into the centre via an external plumbing network, which could be maintained without having to enter the ward; they had buried 200-litre water containers in the ground to store faecal waste and vomit; each bed had a light source above it so that the medical staff could work safely around the clock; and they had security guards around the fence perimeter to prevent disoriented patients from trying to escape. We walked around the outside of the unit. I wasn't allowed inside the centre. Yet somehow, with the help of a few supporting documents, I was supposed to go down to Kenema to recreate it.

MSF had a small team in Kenema that had been sent to bolster the WHO doctors at Kenema Hospital until we could provide more structured assistance. Initially, we planned to build treatment facilities around the hospital to manage Ebola patient overflow and provide clinical support, but when I met with the MSF representative, Elsa, we had to change direction.

I went to sit down on a step near the MSF office, in a far corner of the hospital campus, but Elsa stopped me. She was extremely stressed. 'You can't sit there,' she said. 'Everything is contaminated. There's Ebola everywhere.' We must have been 300 metres from the Ebola ward, but the infection control procedures in the hospital were so bad that the she didn't know for sure that anywhere was safe.

There was a 'no touch' rule between people when it came to Ebola—no handshakes, no hugs, no casual pats on the shoulder—but it very quickly became clear to me that we couldn't touch anything at all. Ebola had a three-week incubation period and we had no idea who was infected at any time, so you had to be extremely vigilant, particularly if you were treating patients. It seemed like this message had failed to sink in at Kenema Hospital. There was no light in the hospital, it was overcrowded and the flow of patient management was poor, but most important, there was no clear delineation between 'red' treatment zones and 'green' safe zones. This went beyond unacceptable to near-suicidal risk, in my opinion.

The WHO doctors were drowning in patients, doing their best to keep up with an unending flow through the hospital doors and putting their own safety at risk as a result. They performed high-risk procedures such as putting central lines into Ebola patients, which presented a huge chance of contamination, while the majority of patients in the ward had neither food nor water. They complained about not having enough nursing staff, as their nursing team was slowly dwindling away. The head matron had died of Ebola, the maternity matron had died of Ebola; in total forty-six members of the hospital staff had been taken by the disease.

The deputy matron at Kenema Hospital was still alive. When I went to visit her to discuss our plans, she sprayed every surface in her office with chlorine before inviting me to sit down. She was remarkably task-oriented and rational, despite what she was dealing with. She agreed with Elsa that it probably wasn't safe for the IFRC to operate in Kenema Hospital and that we should build on a clean site, like MSF had done in Kailahun. They were under enormous pressure from the health department to get Ebola out of Kenema Hospital, and just three days earlier the community had rioted outside, throwing stones and demanding that the Ebola patients be removed.

There was an abandoned airstrip about five kilometres outside of Kenema that would be the perfect site for our treatment centre. There were no houses in the vicinity and the ground was already flat—we could build right on the runway—and because the site was only 5 kilometres from the hospital, we could easily transfer patients. Unfortunately, Sierra Leone's minister of health shut this plan down in its infancy. We wouldn't be allowed to build our hospital within the Kenema city limits.

We were sent to see the local member for parliament, who drove us to another site out along the highway, roughly 17 kilometres from the town. He pointed to a piece of jungle on the side of the road and said, 'You can use as much of this land as you need.'

'I can't build a hospital here,' I told him. 'You need this facility now. Clearing this site will take weeks. We need to build on the airstrip.' He understood, but could only shrug. These decisions were being made at the highest levels of the government.

I fought hard for three or four days, railing against the decision. I fought on the national level, the regional level, and tried to bring international pressure to bear on the situation. Kenema Hospital was cracking under the pressure as more and more patients filled every available corner of the Ebola ward, and the local community was rioting, desperate to have the Ebola clinic moved out of their hospital. The same fear that had ripped through Guinea had taken hold in Sierra Leone and the government's position was clear: 'We cannot guarantee your safety if you build within the city limits.'

I stood my ground, played very tough. We were not going to build a hospital so remote that none of the patients could reach it. But several days after we had visited the site, I received a phone call. On my twelve-dollar Nokia, I heard a woman's voice, 'Please hold for the President of Sierra Leone.'

The line clicked and a very gentle, authoritative voice began to speak. 'Is this Amanda McClelland from the Red Cross?'

'Yes.'

'I would like to thank you and your team for coming to help us in our time of need,' he said. 'I understand you have a problem.'

I leaped at the chance to make my case. The president listened patiently as I worked myself up into a rant. When I was finished, he paused to consider what I had said, and then spoke very calmly. 'Again, I would like to thank you for your offer of assistance'. But he confirmed what the local parliamentarian had told us—that the treatment centre had to be built at the jungle site.

I had a team of foreign IFRC workers arriving in Kenema to build and staff our treatment centre, but nowhere to put them. No hotel in town was interested in housing a group that would be on the frontline in Ebola treatment. Could you blame them? An old friend who I had worked with all the way back in Yirol, a woman named Bridget, was now the Irish Ambassador for Sierra Leone. She made a recommendation: a priest's refectory just outside of town. Late one night, in the belting rain, I went up to see the resident priest, an old Irishman named Father Seamus, who very kindly agreed to host our team for the next couple of weeks, just until we found somewhere else to live. Father Seamus would accommodate the IFRC for the next twelve months.

My architect and civil engineer were two women from the Spanish IFRC, long-term volunteers who deployed regularly with a team of Spanish builders. They were incredibly enthusiastic, a team with a really great attitude, though admittedly I had no idea what they were saying most of the time. The women took one look at our site in the jungle and told me we would need heavy machinery to clear it. Maybe we could engage the Chinese crew that was building the highway out of Kenema?

The highway team was part of China's foreign aid effort, building infrastructure in Sierra Leone, but they hadn't been seen for weeks. They had locked themselves inside their compound when the Ebola outbreak started. I managed to convince them to come out and clear the jungle for us, promising no one would go near them. It took roughly two weeks, but the jungle floor was carnage when they were done. The trees were gone but the rains had come and mud was knee-deep. Half of the land had fallen away. An engineer with the Chinese team said we could probably build on the site in six months.

I went to the local member for parliament and explained that we had tried to do as they asked, but it was impossible. We remained stalled. Meanwhile, a team of IFRC medical staff had now arrived—doctors and nurses from Australia, New Zealand, Norway, England and even Colombia—but without a treatment facility, I was unable to put them to work. This was the peak of the crisis in Kenema—a period in early August where Sierra Leone saw 500–700 new Ebola diagnoses a week. But conditions in the hospital were so poor that it wasn't safe to deploy my team.

There were some phenomenal doctors working at Kenema Hospital. A brilliant infectious diseases specialist had joined the team, an American named Mark, and he did some great work in improving processes at the facility, but every time I saw him he was drenched in sweat and still tried to give me a hug. He was just a very affectionate, personable man, but it was terrifying—staff members at Kenema Hospital were still dying at a disturbing rate. Mark would be infected with Ebola in early September, which resulted in the WHO pulling out of Kenema. He would survive, but there was a wall in Kenema Hospital covered with memorial photos of the staff who didn't.

I had a clinical team in Kenema, but I couldn't send them in to help, not under those conditions. It was incredibly difficult to see so much need and choose not to respond, but I had to be strategic. If one of our expat workers was infected in the first few weeks of the response, there would be no more response. The pressure from foreign governments would shut us down. We had to make sure our team was safe in order to provide the best long-term support.

This meant that our model of care was different to that of the WHO team, which was extremely focused on outcomes for individual patients. They were trying to save lives; we were trying to stop the outbreak. In a situation where cases were overwhelming resources, the focus had to be on staff safety first, then community safety, and finally the individual patients. Once the outbreak was stabilised and we were more experienced, the focus would shift back to patient outcomes. Our model was criticised by some, but in the end I believe it was right.

In the meantime, we needed to find a way to do something. We set up a triage centre outside the grounds of Kenema Hospital to provide more careful sorting of patients. Not everyone with a fever necessarily had Ebola, but if all patients who presented were shoved straight into the Ebola unit, sooner or later they would contract it. Our triage unit lessened a bit of the pressure on the hospital, but the treatment centre was still desperately needed.

A meeting of local government officials, army representatives and other interested parties was called, and together we drove out past the churned-up site that had been cleared by the Chinese, another 2 kilometres down the road to a clearing in the jungle. 'You can build here instead,' I was told.

I was pissed off. We were nearly 20 kilometres from town; how would I get staff to and from the centre? How would patients get to us? We were literally in the middle of the jungle. I threw a very controlled tantrum for the benefit of the assembled committee, but when I was done, the local member took me aside and the message was the same.

'I completely understand what you are saying. I completely agree with you. But this is all we can offer you. You must find a way to make it work.'

I had been in Sierra Leone for almost a month and we still

didn't have an operational treatment centre. People were dying. I had no choice.

Over the next two weeks, the Spanish construction team kicked into gear and I spread my time between the site, coordination meetings and the triage facility at Kenema Hospital. I did daily rounds and kept a close eye on the hospital in particular, because that was the greatest risk to my staff in terms of potential infections. One day, while I was standing outside the triage tent, I saw a boy who was maybe ten years old step through the hospital gate with an older man draped over his shoulder, probably his father. The man staggered forward and fell to the ground just a metre or so in front of me. He was covered in sweat, with blood trickling from his nose. It could have been anything, but it was most likely Ebola.

Within minutes, the man stopped breathing and died.

The media hysteria around Ebola climbed during my first six-week mission to Sierra Leone, which threw up an increasing number of challenges. Kenya shut down all flights from West Africa into the country, which meant we had difficulty shipping in supplies. I had a senior nurse who had worked with me on multiple missions accept a position in the Gaza Strip, where they were literally bombing hospitals, rather than come and work on Ebola. Meanwhile, the international health community was struggling with internal accusations and recriminations, and international governments were dragging their feet when it came to a response.

At Kenema Hospital, the deputy matron held her ground and did an incredible job at getting some infection prevention control protocols in place, ever vigilant. Behind her desk, pinned to the wall, there was a photograph of four nurses; three were women from Sierra Leone, and one was a young Englishman named Simon.

They were holding a baby whose mother had gone into the Ebola ward, though the baby had cleared the 21-day isolation period without showing symptoms. They had taken a shine to the cute little thing and bought him some new clothes from the market, and they were huddled around him in the picture, showing off his new outfit. Every one of them had contracted Ebola. The deputy matron kept the photo as a reminder. They had asked her to be in the photo, but she had refused because it was not safe.

In the middle of all of this, I started to worry about the IFRC teams that were now operating in Guinea and Liberia. Building the hospital had taken much longer than planned and I hadn't had time to analyse in any detail what was happening in the rest of the outbreak. We called a meeting of key personnel to discuss operational strategies, and agreed to hold it in Guinea because the team there couldn't get out; the border was closed. I made the eight-hour drive up towards Guéckédou, glad for the opportunity to see what was happening on the ground. I was also keen to see A——, who was stationed in Guéckédou again.

The passport control office at the border was no bigger than a bathroom, staffed by officials who were extremely friendly—they hadn't seen anyone in weeks—but very uncomfortable about touching our passports. They knew we were working on Ebola. They stamped pieces of paper and handed those to us instead.

At the river crossing into Guinea, we couldn't get the ferry to pick us up. It remained seemingly frozen on the opposite bank, despite the best efforts of the Sierra Leone border guards to radio through to it on our behalf. The border was closed, even for the IFRC. Eventually, I called A——, who called the local police chief in Guéckédou, who drove down and came to our rescue.

My rendezvous with A—— in Guéckédou was totally PG. We sat on opposite ends of the bed with our hands in our laps, just talking. Over the next twelve months, we would both continue to work in Ebola, meeting frequently in different locations around West Africa, in and out of infection zones and quarantine periods. For the better part of twelve months, we didn't touch.

# 20

# IF WE DON'T DO IT, WHO WILL?

My first mission to Sierra Leone ended after six weeks, just before the Kenema treatment centre opened its doors in August 2014. I was called back to Geneva for program oversight, but I would spend the next eight months travelling in and out of West Africa, managing different parts of the IFRC Ebola response.

Overall, the Ebola response was massive. It involved multiple organisations, governments and aid agencies, rolling out across multiple districts in three different countries, each of which had different stakeholders, different challenges and different solutions. I saw everything through the lens of the IFRC, but even that limited view was chaos. We worked so fast that everything became a blur.

There were five pillars in the response effort that had to happen simultaneously in order to contain the outbreak: social mobilisation, case management, contact tracing, dead body management and psychosocial support. Social mobilisation was the education and community awareness program and case management was the isolation of victims in hospitals and treatment centres. There was specific treatment for Ebola, so we did our best to manage people's pain and keep them hydrated, but the primary purpose of those facilities was to stop the disease from spreading. As the outbreak response rolled on, more advanced care and different treatment options were tried, but whether or not patients lived or died seemed to depend on their 'viral load' and without advanced intensive care we were pretty much powerless to affect it—the best we could hope for was a 10-15 per cent reduction in fatalities with good clinical care.

The contact tracing, or chain of transmission tracing, involved making a record of everyone who had come into contact with an infected person and then visiting those people for the next twenty-one days to check if they had developed symptoms. It involved some detective skills, navigating some fear-driven misdirection and lying in the community, but it was absolutely crucial work.

The psychosocial support teams helped communities to deal with the pain of what had happened to them. Along with the terror and the grief, there was a huge amount of survivor's guilt. Some communities lost up to 60 per cent of their people, and some families lost all but one member; the people who survived were left to wonder why they were the lucky ones. People who survived had been through an incredibly traumatic experience in the Ebola wards, watching patients around them suffer horrific deaths and expecting the same for themselves, and afterwards they were returned to a community that would often shun them out of panic, not understanding that they were free of the disease. The psychosocial teams would try to support and help the survivors to reintegrate, while working on other programs that put the feelings of the community first, particularly when it came to dealing with dead bodies.

As we progressed, the Federation changed the name of the dead body management program to 'safe and dignified burials' and worked much harder to involve the community in the process. We had reacted quickly to the initial surge of Ebola and done what we thought was best to contain the disease, but it was a brutal, alienating process for the family and friends of people who had died, which was part of why they'd resisted our intervention. As the response effort progressed, the program was modified so that family members could wear PPE and help with the burial process. At the very least, we brought the bodies out where the community could see and pray for them; we recruited more women into the burial teams, in keeping with local customs; and we brought imams and priests into the burial teams and conducted small ceremonies for the families.

The IFRC had 1500 volunteers managing safe and dignified burials at the peak of the outbreak. Our teams dealt with all the burials in Guinea, half of the burials in Sierra Leone and all the burials in Monrovia, the capital of Liberia. As the outbreak spiralled out of control, it was impossible to know who had died of Ebola and who hadn't. The governments of the three affected countries made an unprecedented decision to bury everyone who died with Ebola precautions, whether or not they had tested positive for the disease. The IFRC teams buried or cremated 46,000 bodies over the course of the outbreak.

At first, the secretary general of the Sierra Leone IFRC had been reluctant to commit his volunteers to the burial program, no matter how hard I tried to convince him that it was essential work and could be done safely. The unsafe burials were driving the outbreak, causing large numbers of infections. Meanwhile, the local IFRC teams had access and the trust of the community that no one else had. It made sense that they did the work, but the secretary general wanted to protect his team. It wasn't just the danger of getting Ebola, it was the stigma the teams would face.

It wasn't until he visited some volunteers who were already at work in Kailahun that he changed his mind. He asked one of the young guys, no more than eighteen, why he had volunteered to pick up the dead bodies. The young man replied, very simply, 'If we don't do it, who will?'

The secretary general came to me and said, 'Tell me what you need us to do.' It changed everything for us.

We needed hundreds of volunteers—at least two hundred staff for the treatment centre, and over fifteen hundred for the burial teams. I wasn't sure we would get the numbers we needed, but so many people stepped forward. At the peak of the emergency we would have over six thousand volunteers active across the three countries that were worst affected, and hundreds more active in the surrounding nations.

The teams were terrified. During the earliest days of training the Kenema treatment centre, I could see their fear. It was completely understandable—most of them were not medically trained. We had a handful of nurses to do clinical care, but the majority of staff would be working on infection prevention and control, cleaning up and providing general care to patients as well as managing the dead. They would see firsthand, day after day, the gruesome reality of an Ebola death, which claimed roughly half the people who came through our doors. It's not just that it was so contagious or killed in such high numbers, it was the way people could die—with severe vomiting, diarrhoea, bleeding, sweats and seizures, untouched by another human being.

The only way to keep 6000 non-medically trained people safe in the deadliest outbreak in the world was to drill them. Many of the volunteers had been active during the long civil wars in Sierra Leone and Liberia, and the younger ones had grown up knowing nothing but conflict. They saw this as a war too. Ebola was the enemy and they would not let their communities be victims. They practised putting on and taking off the PPE for days, and we supervised and observed them for weeks, making sure that they were as safe as they could be. We used the rhetoric of the war against Ebola to marshal them and they rose up to the challenge. Ebola was our mortal enemy. Together, we would fight and we would win.

Beside our volunteers, the unsung heroes of the Ebola response were the logistics teams. We needed 500 LandCruisers in the field at one point. The Federation had a massive car depot in Dubai to support large operations, but it couldn't meet the demand, so we had to negotiate private rentals. We needed PPE kits for the 1500 staff members on burial duty plus the hundreds more staffing our treatment centres, and any given operation would have to stop if we ran out of just one piece of equipment. We also had to mix tonnes and tonnes of chlorine over the course of the response— a highly volatile substance that is classified as a chemical weapon. All of this had to be managed without the usual infrastructure and transport systems that were mobilised in an emergency, as airlines were cancelling services and the region was inaccessible.

The coordination of the response—the command and control centres, the communication across government and aid agencies— was more crucial in the Ebola context than any I had ever seen, because all five pillars of the response effort had to work together in order to be effective. The doctors and nurses got a lot of glory, but the network of people running the operation around them deserved just as much of the credit.

Things changed in September 2014, when the scale of the crisis began to hit home and the rest of the world started to mobilise. By late September, there were more than 6500 diagnosed cases and

3000 deaths from Ebola, including with the first case diagnosed on American soil. Then-president Barack Obama committed 3000 troops to support health operations in West Africa and the British followed within a few weeks with almost 1000 troops. The military brought air support, shipping, infrastructure and security, backing an increased surge in activity from WHO and CDC.

For me, this was sometimes a help, but often a hindrance. My life had become a haze of movement in and out of different countries and different Ebola response programs, as we reacted to different issues, adjusted our strategy and continually expanded our operations. It was easier to function, in some respects, when there were fewer people running around trying to help.

In Monrovia, I was continually putting out fires with stakeholders. The IFRC teams were working in the middle of an urban slum. At the peak of the crisis, the treatment centres were overflowing, unable to absorb the number of patients requiring isolation, and people were dying on the street; the burial teams were collecting bodies in the back of flatbed trucks and taking them to be cremated because there was nowhere to bury them. I was the bad cop standing between the IFRC team and the onslaught of interested parties who always demanded that we do more.

Back in Sierra Leone, the Kenema treatment centre was running well, and we tried to make the patients as comfortable as possible. There was a central part of the ward where patients could convalesce or recover, separated from the green zone by two lines of fencing, with a no-man's-land in between where we could leave things for the patients. They had three meals a day, if they could eat, and all the snacks and drinks they wanted in between those meals. We found coconuts worked best for dehydration, because they were easy to hold—water was served in plastic bags in that part of

Africa, and they were often too hard for the patients to manage. We bought about 300 coconuts every day and I employed a guy whose only job was to cut them open before we passed them out.

There was a little boy named Adam in the ward, about ten years old, who helped us to distribute the coconuts to the other patients. He was recovering quite well from the Ebola infection and had decided that he wanted to become a doctor. One day, Adam was in the lounge area with a group of mothers, one of whom had a very small baby girl who was only seven or eight months old. The baby had Ebola and was not doing well. All we could do was encourage the mother to keep her hydrated. The mother was drip-feeding the baby with coconut milk when she began to have a seizure, convulsing stiffly and frothing at the mouth. The mother panicked, put the child on the floor and ran away crying.

I was only a metre away, behind the safety fence but within reach, unable to help. There were no staff members in the red zone—the last rotation was already in the decontamination area getting undressed. I called to the medical team to put on their PPE and turned back to the baby, and noticed that Adam was still sitting there, frozen. He could only stare at me, paralysed with fear, until the baby died.

The baby had Ebola, it was always going to die, but I still wonder if that little boy felt responsible. The safety protocols meant that we were hamstrung; there was only so much we could do for the patients, which meant they were under this unique pressure to care for each other sometimes. It was a very cruel burden.

How could we make a situation like that seem normal? We did the best we could. We provided board games and cards to keep the patients entertained—things we could then disinfect or throw away. The teams spent hours sitting and talking with patients across the fence, and the local team members sang hymns and songs to encourage the patients to stay motivated, to maintain the will to live when all they wanted to do was die.

We set up Bluetooth speakers in the ward and a projection screen out in the safe zone so that we could screen movies every couple of nights. We bought popcorn at the market, and the patients who were well enough sat eating popcorn and sipping soda while they watched *Toy Story* and *Shrek*. Somehow, sometimes, despite everything that was going on, it felt like an ordinary hospital.

The stigma of working in Ebola was very real. IFRC volunteers were evicted from their accommodation and denied service at restaurants. Families of our staff members relocated children from their homes and went to live with other relatives, and parents told their sons and daughters not to come home.

At one point, two brothers from the Kenema treatment unit were arrested for attempted murder. When I went to try to figure out what had happened, I discovered that the boys' mother had falsified the charges, convinced that they would be safer in jail than working with the IFRC.

The burial teams probably had it worst. They were threatened and even attacked as they tried to collect the dead. Sticks and stones were thrown at their cars. In one Guinean village, a IFRC car was set on fire and the road was barricaded to stop anyone from getting through. A team of high-level officials went in to negotiate with the villagers to try and arrange access for health workers, and eight of the officials were killed, their bodies dumped in a well. The IFRC volunteer who had gone along with them narrowly escaped the same fate.

Despite all this, the teams never wavered. The experience seemed to bring them closer together, some of them even moved in together, and we supported them however we could. We rented houses for some, provided meals at work, hired barbers to cut their hair. We increased our communication with the communities affected by Ebola to try to reduce the risk, and took more time before entering new areas. Still, I worried we were asking too much of them. I had no idea what the long-term impact would be.

Meanwhile, the stigma around working in Ebola wasn't limited to the local staff. When I returned to Geneva after my first trip to Sierra Leone, it was gently suggested that I might be more comfortable working from home. I wasn't allowed to eat my lunch in the cafeteria with the rest of the IFRC. Expats travelling home to Australia were detained in Morocco and were not allowed to board their flights home. After appearing in the media to encourage support for the Ebola response, another Australian nurse was spotted on the beach at home and the police were called. They politely suggested that she leave, for the safety of everyone there.

But if the stigma was real, so were the risks. Everyone who worked in Ebola became hyper-vigilant about monitoring their own health. A sore throat and headache were the first signs of Ebola, but they were also the first signs of almost any viral illness. I would wake up some mornings and before I had even opened my eyes, I would do a mental check. *Is that slight headache? I worked eighteen hours yesterday, I'm probably just tired. Or did I make a mistake somewhere?*

Any sign of fever or illness in any of the staff had to be reported, and the staff member had to be isolated until tests could be done. There were checkpoints all over the affected countries and at international airports where your temperature was taken before you could proceed, and movement was still heavily restricted. On one trip to the airport, I had my temperature taken thirteen times. Inside the affected countries, there were handwashing stations everywhere. You couldn't enter or leave a shop, government building or residency without washing your hands and spraying your feet in chlorine. The stench of chlorine permeated everything. I smelled like a public swimming pool for months.

Despite all the precautions, infection between co-workers happened all too regularly, especially Kenema, a government hospital, where sick nurses had continued to come to work, infecting their colleagues. Altogether, almost 900 health workers would become infected with Ebola over the course of the outbreak, including a number of expats.

In December 2014, we lost a IFRC team member in Guinea. He was a driver who had climbed out the car to make some repairs while there were Ebola patients in the back, had somehow been infected, and died shortly afterwards. It was the first loss we had had, and it bothered me deeply. Within the organisation, we had to consider the possibility that our volunteers were tired, maybe complacent, because they had been working on the outbreak for so long. We would need to re-train everyone—there was no room for complacency.

Things had settled down in Kenema, the peak had well and truly passed, but the treatment centre had started getting a number of referrals from a hospital further north, in Kono. They were coming by ambulance but arriving very late in the day, which wasn't ideal for our team. Working at night increased the risk of infection.

I was in-country, so I decided to investigate, driving up to Kono with a small team from the centre in Kenema. When we arrived, the hospital looked all but deserted, a lifeless, U-shaped cluster of buildings with an overrun garden roundabout in the middle. As we drove around its curve, we saw two dead bodies lying on the hospital steps. 'Stay in the car,' I told the team.

There was red and white police tape wrapped around two pillars, forming a flimsy barricade around the bodies, but no one in sight. It reminded me of Kenema Hospital in the early days of the outbreak. Beyond the two dead bodies, I could see through the hospital doors that there were four or five other patients, clearly very sick with Ebola.

I made my way around the edge of the building and found another ward, full of sick children who were obviously not Ebola patients, but still no staff. I kept walking, and eventually found an office with two American doctors inside.

'Hi,' I said.

'Hello, how are you?'

'My name is Amanda McClelland and I'm from the IFRC treatment centre in Kenema. You guys have been referring Ebola patients to us. I'm looking for someone called Dr Sam?' This was the only information we had been given by the referred patients—Dr Sam had sent them.

'Hi, I'm Sam,' said one of the men, reaching his hand out to shake mine. *What the fuck.* I hadn't shaken anyone's hand in months.

'Uh, that's okay,' I politely declined. My hands remained, as usual, in my pockets. 'So what's going on?'

'We're just getting ready to go into the Ebola ward.'

'Pardon?'

There was no one to spray them down, no green zone, they were just going to throw their PPE on and walk through the entire hospital to the Ebola ward and then when they came out, I don't know . . . undress in their office? Sam had a pair of pliers in his hand, with which he was going to cut down some infected mosquito nets in the ward.

'Hey, do you guys need some help here?' I asked.

'Yeah, that would really be great.'

These two doctors were part of a development program attached to an American university that regularly sent medical staff to the hospital in Kono. They had been helping the ministry of health to manage Ebola in the district but they were clearly under-resourced for the activity. Nine of the nurses from the ministry had died of Ebola the week before we arrived and the rest of the team had run away. Frankly, I was astounded that these two hadn't been infected.

'We're doing everything we can until help arrives,' they told me.

Negotiations were underway for another aid organisation to come in and build an Ebola treatment centre, but the doctors were hazy on the details. There was no firm date. They didn't have the funding. I told them I could send a team up the next day to at least establish a triage centre, but it wasn't in their power to say *yes, go ahead.*

'How about the dead bodies out there, are you going to do something with them?'

The doctors couldn't manage it, so I had my team suit up in their PPE and deal with the corpses on the steps. Ultimately, I had to set up a triage unit in Kono just to ensure the safety of my staff in Kenema. If we could control the flow of patients and make sure they were coming down to us in better condition, the risk of things going wrong was that much less. Within three days, we were set up outside. We had also cleaned and secured the Kono Ebola ward and convinced some of the Kono nursing staff to come back so that the rest of the hospital was operational.

Unfortunately, things didn't run smoothly. There were complications, politics, and differences of opinion about the patient referral process which led to unsafe conditions back in Kenema, and further risks to our staff. We needed more control. I had the funds and equipment to build a full treatment centre in Kono, but the hospital wanted the IFRC to build it in partnership with another aid organisation and that didn't work for us. We had to be able to implement our protocols and our procedures to ensure safety for our staff. I held firm. We wouldn't partner inside the red zone. Eventually, they asked us to do it alone.

The Spanish team that had built the Kenema facility came back to build the treatment centre in Kono, and they did it in record time. They were an amazing team—no challenge too big—and worked right through Christmas without complaint.

On New Year's Eve, the flow of patients from Kono reached a peak. We had eighty-three patients in the unit, with another fifteen on their way, and I went in to the centre to check on the teams and make sure they could handle it. I spent most of my time on the phone, not caring for patients, so I was glad to be back in the centre even for a little while.

As 2014 ticked in 2015, I found myself wrangling a delirious Ebola patient. She was naked and stalking the ward for people with a suspected but unconfirmed Ebola infection, carrying a dirty adult diaper in her hand. The woman was threatening to throw her nappy at patients who had symptoms, but had yet to test positive for the virus. I had to tackle her and throw her over my shoulder while another nurse gave her a sedative shot. I don't know if it was a happy new year, but it certainly was a memorable one.

By mid-January 2015, the treatment centre in Kenema was virtually empty, as was the centre in Kono. The medical teams saw febrile patients, but it was rarely Ebola. And while the burial teams were still working, it was largely precautionary, as the bodies only rarely tested positive for Ebola. The end of the crisis was still several months away, but the peak was well and truly over.

I was due to head back to Geneva—I was done—but I had stopped to work with the team in Monrovia, to help them move into the recovery phase. Schools had shut down during the outbreak; much of the agrarian activity had stopped; pregnant women hadn't had access to medical care. The repercussions of the outbreak ran so deeply in the community that it would take a long time just to understand their scope, but what we could see, we could try to fix. There was no shortage of things to do.

While I was in Liberia, I received a phone call to say that one of the nurses at the Kenema treatment centre had died. I had just left there; I hadn't even known he was sick. We had a unit to monitor staff health and the nurse had been brought in, but he had died within twenty minutes of arrival. They had tested for Ebola, but they thought he had died of cardiac failure. When the test results came back, they were positive.

Two of the expat doctors had treated the nurse before he died. The local staff had taken bloods and put a catheter in the sick man, and urine had spilled on the floor. They weren't wearing PPE. All up, there were about twenty staff members involved. Maybe after so many months without an incident people had become complacent, I don't know. Perhaps they all just trusted each other too much.

I jumped in a car and drove ten hours from Monrovia down to Kenema. When I arrived, the team leader was still on his feet; he hadn't slept for a couple of days. He was sorry, he said, but he needed to go. He left for Freetown for a day's rest, but didn't come back for another three days. Meanwhile, I was left to figure out what had happened and who else was infected. The district medical officer was ropable because we had started a new chain of infection in Kenema, when the district had been clear for several weeks. Clinically, personally, it was just a nightmare. There was something really heavy about the timing. It had felt like the finish line was in sight, and suddenly there was this epic failure. The scrutiny from WHO, CDC and the Sierra Leone ministry of health was incredible.

The story was complicated, but the staff had had a number of reasons to think that the nurse was no danger to them, not least a medical certificate from Kenema Hospital that said he was Ebola-free. The man had been sick for seven days, but had done his best to conceal it. He was very likely in denial. It was difficult to blame him or the team.

I had two expat doctors evacuated. Luckily, neither of them were sick. And eighteen staff put under quarantine while we waited to see if anyone would get sick. The mother of the nurse got sick and died; his sister got sick but survived. Our staff health nurse and the driver who had collected the man also got sick, and they also survived. By some minor miracle, there was no one else. But there was a huge investigation into the incident. I spent days with external agencies, probing the protocols, trying to figure out what went wrong, but there were no obvious breaches to indicate where the original infection had come from.

While I was working through this, I was at the treatment centre, double-checking everything, testing and retesting the safety protocols to make sure the centre was secure. It was the most stress I had felt throughout the entire outbreak. One day, just after we had buried the nurse, I was standing in the green zone watching the infection prevention and control team working inside the red zone. The centre was completely empty, not a single patient, so the team inside the ward was cleaning up. As I watched, one of the guys reached his entire gloved hand into a medical sharps bin.

'What the fuck are you doing?!' I bellowed.

The man froze, staring at me through his PPE goggles, totally confused.

'Just stop. Stop,' I told him. 'Very slowly, very carefully, take your hand out of the container. Okay, now go to the decontamination area and wait for me. I'll be right there.'

I walked away, my hands clasped over the back of my head, not sure if I was going to scream or cry. After the nurse's death, after the scrutiny and recriminations, I'd witnessed something so horrifyingly, basically wrong that it threw my whole sense of control out of the window.

In the decontamination room, I made the staff member fill his gloves with water and squeeze them, to see if there were any punctures. The water held—there were no holes. He didn't have a needle stick injury. I was only mildly relieved.

'Jesus Christ, what would make you put your hand inside a sharps container?' I asked. I was convinced we would have to shut the whole centre down.

'Well, normally we seal the containers and incinerate them,' the man answered. 'But today the doctor told me to empty the containers.'

The doctor he referred to spoke English as a second language. The staff member spoke English as a second language. What word had the doctor meant to use? Empty, clear, destroy, dispose of . . .? Just a stupid little misunderstanding, and the whole thing could have started all over again.

In the end, Ebola took up two years of my life. I left Sierra Leone early in 2015 but the work and support from the office in Geneva continued for another year, and it was all-consuming. The WHO released statistics in May 2015—there had been 27,000 Ebola cases and around 11,000 deaths—but the cases stuttered on over the months, never quite vanishing completely, and the crisis work evolved to recovery work, which is ongoing.

During those critical two years, other things happened, unrelated things, but for A— and me it was a blur of urgency, crisis, putting out fires and trying to predict where we would be needed next. If my partner hadn't been as dedicated to the response as I was, I may not have been so deeply involved. We enabled each other and supported each other to constantly re-submerge ourselves in the emergency, and it changed us, both professionally and personally. When we talk about our lives now, there is a clear demarcation—before and after Ebola.

I learned an incredible amount through the experience, especially about myself. I had been arrogant and too direct at times, which was a bad move politically. But I've thought about it and I struggle to see how it could have been done differently. We had to move so fast, against such a heavy tide of resistance, misunderstanding and complacency, and I was fighting very hard as a nurse and as a health advisor to stop the disease from spreading.

I was proud of many of the things we achieved, and how quickly we achieved them, but when I think back on my most successful missions, Ebola is not one of them. For some of the expats who worked with us, Ebola would be their first and last mission; it was just too traumatic. Some of the local staff struggled to return to normal life. They were in steady jobs for a long time, then the work suddenly dried up. After spending a year collecting dead bodies, they were not always welcomed back with open arms to their family or their community. And the scars that were left in the community because of the disease, because of the well-intended but fumbling nature of the initial response, were too deep to even comprehend. We didn't leave the people, the communities or their health systems more robust than we had found them, and that was a very uncomfortable feeling for me.

Having said that, I would do it again. I would do it better. And we will have to do it again, it's just a matter of time.

# EPILOGUE

Okay so maybe the title is a bit misleading—my experience is a little broader than emergencies only. In my career, I've been an educator, an engineer, a project manager, a negotiator and a consultant. I've travelled all over the world and dealt with all kinds of health issues and emergencies, from minor cuts to global catastrophes. Some of it may seem heroic, but it's not. It's a job. I found a career that I was good at it and I stuck with it, and this is where I ended up.

Every step of the way, I had a little more training, I gained a little more experience and I kept studying, until I became a highly skilled humanitarian worker. But fundamentally, I'm interested in the same thing now that interested me at the start of my career—public health. I will always think of myself as a paediatric nurse, first and foremost, because nursing and healthcare are at the heart of everything I do. As far as I'm concerned I'm just a nurse, but that's not how other people see it.

I spend a lot of time on planes, normally on the way to or from a disaster zone, generally beyond exhausted or focused on what comes next. I am not a big fan of small talk in this situation. I like the twenty-four hours of alone time I get with long-haul, even if it is in cattle class—no emails, no phone calls and no big decisions. I can go almost a full day where the only choice I have to make is between chicken or fish. But if I don't get my headphones on fast enough, if the person sitting next to me feels like a chat, the conversation that follows is often painfully awkward for me.

'Where are you headed?' they ask. My answer is rarely typical. 'Where is that?' they want to know, 'And why are you going there?'

When I explain what I do for a living, a certain type of person tells me they've always wanted to do some humanitarian work. How can they get involved? For these people, 'humanitarian' is code for a glamorous career where you save a poor African, meet a handsome human rights lawyer and then retire. You live happily ever after, somewhere in Europe, safe in the knowledge that you once spent six months trying to save the world.

Other people say, 'You must see some terrible things!' and look at me like my dog was just run over. Their expression is a mixture of pity and intrigue, an expression that is asking for details. *How horrible is it, exactly? Tell me all the gory details.* They want to know how nobly I have suffered, and when I'm done, they want to thank me for doing my job, like a payment for services rendered on their behalf. I hate to disappoint these people, but I really love what I do.

Yes, I've seen some terrible things. People are at their most vulnerable in poverty, crisis and conflict. A disaster can knock a community to its knees and do some lasting damage. But I arrive to provide relief, so the first thing I usually experience is gratitude. I see community spirit, resilience and people's desire to live a good life, despite the horrible things that have happened to them. I see people doing their best when it really counts; caring for each other, lifting each other up and making each other laugh. It's not all doom and gloom. And anyway, I always remember the funniest stories best.

I laugh a lot when I think about where I have been and the things I have done. Ultimately, that's why I decided to write this book. I'm not philosophical. I'm no expert on the impact of colonialism on global poverty or the failures of the aid dollar. I don't lose sleep over the horrible decisions I have been forced to make because I couldn't save every life and I am not the aid worker that moved to Africa and fell in love with a Zulu warrior only to realise the harsh realities of life in a mud hut. I'm a nurse, I'm a humanitarian, and I had a few good stories to tell. I hope that you enjoyed them.

# Acknowledgements

I would like to thank the many people who made this book possible.

Simone Ubaldi and her dog George, who battled through conflicting travel schedules, time zones and bad Skype connections to capture the humanity, complexity and humour of the situations I have found myself in over the last twenty years.

The many people who read and gave feedback on various parts of the book. Thank you, you know who you are.

The Australian Red Cross for its support in both my career as a humanitarian and in helping me to share the stories of the work that we do together.

All of my colleagues and the communities that we work with and for.

My friends and family. It is true that this career is hardest on those who stay behind, but you have been supportive no matter what path I have chosen.

And my partner. This work can be lonely, and hard to understand. I am grateful I have found someone who shares my passion, drive and dreams, but most importantly understands that when I get excited about an outbreak of monkeypox, it's because it's interesting, not because I am weird.